N

Nurse

For Elsevier:

Associate Editor: Mairi McCubbin
Project Manager: Jess Thompson
Typesetting and Production: Helius
Cover Design: Kneath Associates

New Practice Nurse

Edited by

Julia Lucas MSc RGN General Practice Specialist Nurse

Practice Nurse Manager, Rosedean Surgery, Liskeard, Cornwall, UK

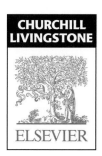

Edinburgh   London   New York   Oxford   Philadelphia   St Louis   Sydney   Toronto   2007

CHURCHILL
LIVINGSTONE
ELSEVIER

An imprint of Elsevier Limited

First published 2007

ISBN-10: 0 443 10261 9
ISBN-13: 978 0 443 10261 5

British Library Cataloguing in Publication Data
A catalogue record for this book is available from the British Library

Library of Congress Cataloging in Publication Data
A catalog record for this book is available from the Library of Congress

Notice
Knowledge and best practice in this field are constantly changing. As new research and experience broaden
our knowledge, changes in practice, treatment and drug therapy may become necessary or appropriate.
Readers are advised to check the most current information provided (i) on procedures featured or (ii) by the
manufacturer of each product to be administered, to verify the recommended dose or formula, the method and
duration of administration, and contraindications. It is the responsibility of the practitioner, relying on their
own experience and knowledge of the patient, to make diagnoses, to determine dosages and the best treatment
for each individual patient, and to take all appropriate safety precautions. To the fullest extent of the law,
neither the Publisher nor the Editor assumes any liability for any injury and/or damage to persons or property
arising out of or related to any use of the material contained in this book.

The Publisher

Working together to grow
libraries in developing countries

www.elsevier.com | www.bookaid.org | www.sabre.org

ELSEVIER BOOK AID
International Sabre Foundation

ELSEVIER your source for books,
journals and multimedia
in the health sciences
www.elsevierhealth.com

The
publisher's
policy is to use
**paper manufactured
from sustainable forests**

Printed in Spain

Contents

Contributors

Gilly Andrews RGN
Menopause Nurse Specialist, Lister Hospital,
London

Kirsty Armstrong SRN FPCert BSc(Hons) NP Dip
Senior Lecturer and Primary Care Practitioner,
Faculty of Health and Social Care Sciences,
St. George's Hospital Medical School, Kingston
University; Nurse Practitioner, London

Maureen Benbow MSc BA RGN HERC
Tissue Viability Nurse, Mid Cheshire Hospital
Trust, Crewe

Tina Bishop BSc(Hons) MA DipN PGCE RGN
Senior lecturer, Anglia Polytechnic University,
Chelmsford

Rachel Booker RGN DN(Cert) HV
Head of Student Support, National Respiratory
Training Centre, Warwick

Sue Clarke BSc(Hons) RGN RHV SPPH DN NP
Senior Child and Family Nurse, South
Cambridgeshire PCT; Nurse Adviser to the
Anaphylaxis Campaign

Maggie Cooper RGN DipN
Practice Nurse Trainer, Surrey; Breast and
Cervical Screening Courses Adviser, Marie Curie
Cancer Care

Jane DeVille-Almond SRN SCM HV BA(Hons)
Independent Nurse Consultant, Wolverhampton

Bridgit Dimond MA LLB DSA AHSM
Barrister-at-law; Emeritus Professor, University
of Glamorgan

Carolyn Driver MSc RGN RM RHV FPCert
Travel health specialist; Chair of the British
Travel Health Association, Sale

Simon Ebbett
News Editor, *Doctor*

Gwen Hall RMN RGN BSc(Hons)
Diabetes Specialist Nurse in Primary Care and
Practice Nurse, Guildford and Waverley PCT

Keith Hampton MA BSc(Hons) RGN
Nurse Consultant in Infection Control, Havering
PCT, Hornchurch

Hilary Harkin RGN BSc(Hons)
Trainer in Primary Ear Care and ENT Nurse
Practitioner, Guy's and St. Thomas' Hospitals,
London

Victoria Harmer RN BSc(Hons) Dip(Breast Care)
MBA AKC
Clinical Nurse Specialist, Breast Care, St. Mary's
Hospital, London

Sharon Harris RGN
Sister, Dialysis Unit, Ashford Hospital, part of
the Hammersmith Hospital Renal Unit, London

Ken Hines MD
General Practitioner, South Woodford; PEC
member, Redbridge PCT; accredited Immediate
Care Practitioner; founder member of the British
Association for Immediate Care (BASICS)

Briony Ladbury RGN RM HV FPnurse BA(Hons)
Interprofessional Studies (Protecting Children),
ENB Specialist Practitioner Child Protection,
Designated Nurse in Child Protection and Child
Protection Manager, Croydon PCT

Mike McGhee LRCP MRCS MB BS MRCGP
DRCOG MFFP DOccMed
General Practitioner, Castle Donington, Derby;
GP Trainer, Nottingham GP Vocational Training

Sue Nutbrown RGN RM DipN BA(Hons)
MMedSci
Practice Nurse and Primary Care Nurse Adviser,
Sheffield; Chair of the RCN Practice Nurse
Association, London

Jennifer Percival RGN RM HVCert
Tobacco Education Project Manager, Royal
College of Nursing, London

Nicola Stevens RGN
Respiratory Liaison Nurse (Specialist Nurse) and
Clinical Skills Trainer (ECG), Ninewells Hospital,
Dundee, Tayside Universities NHS Trust

Catriona Sutherland
Clinical Nurse Specialist in Contraception and
Sexual Health, Paxton Green Group Practice,
South London

Steven Walker MD
Medical Writer

Nerys Williams MBCHS MRCGP FFOM FRCP
Consultant Occupational Physician, Birmingham;
Honorary Consultant in Obesity/Weight
Management, Birmingham Heartlands and
Solihull NHS Trust, Birmingham

Preface

General Practice continues to evolve and, alongside it, Practice Nursing. The New General Medical Service Contract, Practice Based Commissioning and Primary Care Trust reconfiguration all mean that the Practice Team requires an increasingly greater skill mix. It is hoped that this book will give nurses new to General Practice Nursing knowledge of some of the initial core skills needed. Each chapter is written by an expert in that field and contains a wealth of information. The chapters were originally published as articles in *Practice Nurse* journal.

Julia Lucas

Section 1

Health promotion and health education

SECTION CONTENTS

Chapter 1

Childhood immunization and vaccination

Kirsty Armstrong

CHAPTER CONTENTS

Immunization has been around for over 1,000 years, when the Chinese first inoculated people against smallpox by grinding dried smallpox pustules into a powder and blowing it into their noses, which produced immunity after a mild illness.[1]

In the UK protection against smallpox started in the 18th century with Edward Jenner and the milkmaid inoculated with cowpox. Immunization against infectious diseases has reduced mortality and morbidity over the years but with the disappearance of these diseases it becomes more difficult to explain the advantages.

The principles of immunization are to protect individuals from disease, prevent outbreaks and eventually eradicate some diseases worldwide. As a new practice nurse you may find that one of the questions that you are asked most is: 'Surely if these diseases are no longer around I don't have to vaccinate my child?'

HERD IMMUNITY

For the majority to be protected against a disease a certain percentage of that population must be able to withstand infection. Immunity from exposure to the disease and from vaccines are both examples of active immunity.

Immunity can also be passed from mother to child *in utero* and during breastfeeding, or from the administration of ready-made antibodies in the form of immunoglobulins (e.g. rabies immunoglobulin for post-exposure protection) – these are both forms of passive immunity.

Figures published by the Public Health Laboratory Service (PHLS) illustrate the impact of falling vaccination:[2] in March 2001 only 83.6% of children nationally had received their first MMR vaccination by their second birthday; herd immunity for measles is estimated at a vaccination rate of 95%. One result of this was an outbreak of 23 cases of measles in a south-west London nursery. Similarly, the Republic of Ireland notified 1,200 cases of measles in 2000, resulting in two deaths, after immunization coverage there dropped to 74.4%.

THE CHILDHOOD SCHEDULE

Table 1.1 shows the current UK schedule, which is included in all the health promotion material available for you to give to parents and promotional posters for the surgery.[2] There are many different schedules around the world and it is not always possible to streamline all children onto the UK schedule.[1] Advice from your colleagues or a telephone call to your local District Immunization Coordinator (DIC) can help with this and can also help you to establish the best way forward in the case of unimmunized children who need vaccination.

In difficult cases be aware of your limitations and defer to those in the know; although they are sometimes hard to get hold of it is better to persevere than make a catastrophic and irrevocable mistake.[2] The PHLS website has a good page with a schedule for unimmunized individuals or those unsure of their vaccinations.[2]

THE COLD CHAIN AND STORAGE OF VACCINES

A protocol will help you to establish whether a vaccine has been stored correctly from the time of its manufacture up until when you administer it. This should include:

- the type of refrigerator used for vaccine storage, which should be a pharmacy fridge with an inbuilt maximum–minimum thermometer
- the temperature at which most vaccines should be stored (see Box 1.1)
- the person responsible for receiving and checking the vaccines and their deputy; this

TABLE 1.1 The current UK childhood schedule		
Age	**Immunization**	**Method of administration**
2, 3 and 4 months	Diphtheria, tetanus, pertussis (whooping cough), polio and Hib (DTaP/IPV/Hib)	One injection
	MenC	One injection
Approximately 13 months	Measles, mumps and rubella (MMR)	One injection
3 years and 4 months to 5 years	Diphtheria, tetanus, pertussis (whooping cough) and polio (DTaP/IPV or DTaP/IPV)	One injection
	Measles, mumps and rubella (MMR)	One injection
10 to 14 years (shortly after birth in exceptional circumstances)	BCG (against tuberculosis)	Skin test then, if needed, one injection
13 to 18 years	Diphtheria, tetanus and polio (Td/IPV)	One injection

BOX 1.1 Correct vaccine storage temperatures	
2–8°C	**0–4°C**
• Pertussis	• Polio
• Diphtheria	• Influenza
• Tetanus	• Hepatitis A
• Hib	• Hepatitis B
• Rabies	• Yellow fever
• MMR	• Typhoid
• Rubella	• Meningitis
• BCG	

should be you as practice nurse and a trained receptionist or colleague.[3]

Most surgeries have vaccines delivered in refrigerated vans by a distribution company, although some, particularly travel vaccines, are sent by post. You must take note of the postmark and if it is more than 48 hours ago contact the manufacturer or distributor as you may need to return or discard the vaccines. Always talk to the company first, otherwise you may be financially accountable. Vaccines should be checked for damage and rotated according to expiry dates.

The ideal fridge temperature is 2–8°C, which should be monitored and recorded every day if possible. Variations around this temperature should be reported to the manufacturers for information about diminished efficacy.

Vaccines are most likely to be damaged by freezing and often develop sediment or clouding as a result. Vaccines left out on desks in warm rooms or repeatedly taken out of the fridge may also lose efficacy.

CONTRAINDICATIONS TO VACCINES

There are three absolute contraindications to vaccine administration – acute febrile illness, pregnancy and severe local or systemic reaction to a preceding dose of the same vaccine.

Immunosuppression is a contraindication with live vaccines such as MMR, BCG, oral polio, oral typhoid and yellow fever, and there should be an interval of at least 3 weeks between vaccines except when polio and BCG are given within the childhood schedule.

When in doubt consult your colleagues, the *British National Formulary* (BNF) or the 'Green Book'.[4]

CONSENT

Remember that you are accountable and liable to obtain informed consent for all the vaccines that you administer so it is a good idea to know what you are giving and why.[2]

You must ascertain how fit the child is to have the vaccine by assessing their health on the day and considering any recent illness or reaction to a previous vaccine. Use this discussion to impart information on what to do if the child develops a raised temperature. Four-hourly paracetamol liquid dosed according to age is advised, but if the fever has not settled after 48 hours or there are worrying symptoms (continuous crying, unusual swelling) further review may be needed.

You may also wish to give information about your local walk-in centre, GP on-call service, NHS Direct helpline and local paediatric casualty department if the vaccine is given before the weekend.

The issue of the caregiver being able to give consent is also paramount – it is only the mother that can always give consent unless parental responsibility has been removed. Others may not be aware of previous problems, know what to do in a crisis or be able to give legal consent.

General issues on informed consent are covered in Chapter 31.

ANAPHYLAXIS

You need to have an annual update on CPR and anaphylaxis and you also need to have an anaphylaxis pack with up-to-date adrenalin in your room at the time of vaccination.

Talk to other practitioners and the receptionists in your surgery and develop a protocol of what to do in an emergency. For example:

- Have you got an emergency bell in your room?
- Whom would you contact?
- Is there oxygen in the practice and where is it located?

Anaphylactoid reactions are rare but babies sometimes go into mild shock (pale and quiet – no crying), which can be as worrying as the babies who cry loud and long. If in doubt ask a colleague to come in and check with you.

PATIENT GROUP DIRECTIONS (PGDs)

Your local PCT training and development coordinator or practice nurse development leader should have PGDs covering all childhood and travel immunizations. You must follow the PGDs to the letter for your action to be legal because you are administering prescription-only medicines to patients without prescriptions. These PGDs are drafted and finalized by your GP, PCT, medical director and lead pharmacist and will list the indications and contraindications for vaccines with various follow-up and review policies. If you are unable to access these documents or your GP says this is not necessary, contact your union or the MDU. Until we are able to prescribe from the BNF we need PGDs to administer vaccinations.

COMMON CONCERNS ABOUT VACCINATIONS

Parents have many concerns about immunizing their children that the practice nurse may have to address.

OVERLOAD OF THE IMMUNE SYSTEM

Many vaccinations are given at the same time; a common worry is overload of the immune system.

However, when you consider the amount of bacteria and viruses children encounter every day through inhalation, putting objects into their mouths and foodstuffs (Is that banana sterile!), concern about using multiple vaccinations fades into insignificance.[5]

RISKS VERSUS BENEFITS

Another common worry is that the risk posed by the vaccines may outweigh that of the disease. The vaccines produced today give the maximum amount of immunity using the smallest amount of attenuated disease.

The false belief that improved hygiene and living conditions preclude the need for protection against disease is borne out by the recent measles outbreak in south-west London – an area that boasts a high standard of living.

Of course the MMR vaccine has recently attracted much media coverage – suffice it to say the evidence still shows there is no link between autism, bowel disease and the MMR. Check the official websites for information for your parents.

INJECTION TECHNIQUE AND NEEDLE LENGTH

This is of vital importance to immunization, but is discussed in a separate chapter. Also consider safe disposal of sharps and potential crisis management.

LATEST INFORMATION

Pneumovax is already part of the regular schedule in the USA and, although in the UK it is currently administered to those in at-risk categories, it will be added into the schedule in summer 2006. Varicella is also part of the USA schedule. The new guidance on DtaP/Hib is to give the Hib at a different site from the DtaP if that is all you have – but wherever possible give the whole-cell pertussis (DTwP).

FURTHER TRAINING

There is no substitute for a good immunization course. If there is one in your area identify it as vital rather than optional. Some PCTs have an induction pathway for new practice nurses of which this forms a part. Updates are also useful.

ESSENTIAL SKILLS
• Consent/legal issues • Contraindications and indications • PGDs • Cold chain • Technique/administration/disposal

REFERENCES

1. Kassianos GC. Immunisation: Childhood and Travel Health, 4th edn. Oxford: Blackwell Science, 2001.
2. Nursing and Midwifery Council. Code of Professional Conduct. London: Nursing and Midwifery Council, 2002: item 6.2, p8.
3. Scade C. A protocol for storing vaccines effectively. Practice Nurse 1999; 17: 387–91.
4. Department of Health. Immunisation Against Infectious Diseases. London: HMSO, 1996. [Also available online at http://www.dh.gov.uk]
5. Offitt PA, Quarles J, Gerber MA, et al. Addressing parents' concerns: do multiple vaccines overwhelm or weaken the infant's immune system? Pediatrics 2002; 109(1): 124–129.

FURTHER READING

Vaccine Administration Taskforce UK. Guidance on Best Practice in Vaccine Administration. London: Shire Hall, 2001.

USEFUL WEBSITES

COVER (Coverage of Vaccinations Evaluated Rapidly) statistics: http://www.phls.co.uk

Department of Health: http://www.dh.gov.uk

Farillon Pharmaceutical Distribution: http://www.farillon.co.uk

Nursing & Midwifery Council: http://www.nmc-uk.org

Chapter 2

Travel vaccination

Carolyn Driver

It can be very daunting when you receive your first request for travel advice from a patient, especially as holiday destinations are becoming more exotic. Where do you start, and from where should you get your information in order to give the best advice? This chapter looks at the basics and some of the more commonly used vaccines.

THE TRAVEL HEALTH CONSULTATION

The advice and vaccinations that you may need to give to your patients do not depend entirely on their destination. You need to conduct a thorough risk assessment and make use of appropriate resources, in order to give sufficient information to help patients make the right choices about preventive interventions. The most important issue is to ensure you have enough time – travel health consultations need to be at least 20 minutes for an individual and longer for a couple or family group. Follow-up appointments can be shorter depending on the requirements of the individual.

THE RISK ASSESSMENT

This needs to include details of the patient's departure date, destination (or destinations if touring, including any overnight stopovers), type of accommodation, duration and purpose of visit, including all likely activities.

The patient's age should be obtained along with details about general health, any chronic or recent medical conditions, medications and vaccination history. Once this information has been established, health education issues and any recommended vaccinations can be discussed. Depending on the destination, malaria prevention may also need to be covered.

INFORMATION SOURCES

There are two basic texts that every surgery should have: the 'Green Book' and the 'Yellow Book'. The Green Book or *Immunisation Against Infectious Disease*, although published in 1996, is still the definitive guide to immunization from the Department of Health (DoH). It can now also be accessed via the DoH's website, where updates continue to be added – so this source should be checked regularly.

Nurses should also ensure that any updates on immunization sent out by the Chief Medical and Nursing Officers are passed on to them and filed along with the Green Book. The Yellow Book or *Health Information for Overseas Travel* is the DoH's principal source of guidance for travellers and is also available on the internet, where it is updated. For details of this and other useful reference sources see the Further Reading section at the end of this chapter.

It is most important that, before administering vaccines to anyone, the nurse should thoroughly familiarize himself or herself with the products to be used by reading the summary of product characteristics (SPC) that is enclosed with all vaccines.

Nurses should also ensure that they are working within the patient group directions that have been drawn up in their area of employment.

The medical information departments of each of the vaccine manufacturers will also talk to healthcare professionals if they have any queries about their products. The company website or the address list in MIMS are the most convenient ways of obtaining contact information.

VACCINATIONS

It is important that the appropriate vaccinations are recommended to travellers. However, there are a number of points the nurse needs to convey to his or her patients:

- vaccination can only prevent 5% of travel-related illness
- coronary heart disease and trauma are the major causes of death in British travellers abroad
- the infections most likely to affect the traveller are the more mundane travellers' diarrhoea or respiratory infections
- the traveller's activities and behaviour abroad are more significant risk factors than simply their destination.[1]

For most destinations there are no compulsory vaccinations, so it is a matter of assessing risk and informing the traveller of the potential hazards, available vaccines and their side-effects, and then allowing the patient to make informed choices. The Yellow Book gives a good explanation of how to assess such risks. The most up-to-date resource a nurse can use to facilitate this process is the online database TRAVAX (see Useful Websites at the end of this chapter). This contains a wealth of information about individual countries as well as background information about specific diseases and different types of traveller. There is a public access version called *Fit for Travel* that is useful to recommend to travellers if they wish to have more information or are unsure about their travel plans. A new helpline has also been set up by the National Travel Health Network and Centre (NaTHNaC) to help with difficult travel queries (telephone 020 7380 9234).

ROUTINE VACCINATIONS AND BOOSTERS

A travel consultation is an ideal time to check that the patient has completed their primary course of routine vaccinations. Particular attention should be paid to people born before the national vaccination programme was introduced in 1960.

Tetanus, diphtheria and polio boosters may be required by those travelling to developing countries for prolonged periods. Diphtheria boosters were introduced to the school leaver's programme in 1994, and if a tetanus booster is required by anyone born before 1979 a combined tetanus, low-dose diphtheria and polio vaccine should be administered. Those who travel frequently to endemic areas should receive boosters every 10 years. Polio has been eradicated from large parts of the world, but all travellers should ensure they have completed a primary course, and boosters are advised for those travelling to sub-Saharan Africa, India, Russia and the former Soviet states.[2]

COMMONLY RECOMMENDED TRAVEL VACCINES

Hepatitis A

Hepatitis A is a food- and water-borne infection, endemic throughout the world. Vaccination is recommended for travellers to any destination outside western Europe, the USA, or Australasia. Inactivated hepatitis A vaccination is very effective and can be administered to patients over 1 year old. It confers a minimum of 10 years' immunity after the complete course.

Schedule

The primary dose is administered by intramuscular injection followed by a booster 6–12 months later. Havrix Junior should be used for those aged 1–15 years; VAQTA Paediatric is licensed for ages 2–17 years. If the booster is delayed it will still produce an antibody response and thus the course need not be restarted, but travellers should be encouraged to attend promptly for their booster in order to ensure continuous protection from the infection.[3] A recall system can help. As the natural infection has an average 4-week incubation period it is always worth offering vaccination even to late presenters.

Typhoid

Typhoid can be transmitted through contaminated food and water. Risk is highest in areas where water supplies may be contaminated with sewage. In some countries vegetables are fertilized with human waste (night soil), and thus if not washed and cooked thoroughly would be sources of infection. Most cases imported to the UK originate in the Indian subcontinent.[4]

Typhoid Vi polysaccharide is an inactivated vaccine that confers about 80% immunity that lasts for 3 years. However, the importance of taking precautions with food and water must be emphasized as the vaccine is only 70–80% protective. This type of vaccine does not produce a good response in children under 2 years of age.

Yellow fever

Yellow fever is a viral illness transmitted to man by the mosquito. The disease is endemic in 33 countries in sub-Saharan Africa and ten countries in tropical South America. It is the only remaining vaccination to carry an International Certificate of Vaccination under international health regulations.

The aim is to stop the spread of infection to countries where it is currently not endemic, and consequently the strictest regulations exist where travellers are entering a non-infected country from an endemic area. The Yellow Book gives further information on this issue. The vaccine is a live attenuated vaccine that confers long-term immunity after just one dose. It should be administered by deep subcutaneous injection and can be used from 9 months of age.

Although evidence suggests that the vaccine confers significantly longer immunity, the WHO regulations advocate revaccination after 10 years for those at potential risk or who require certificates.[5] Individuals travelling to countries where there is a certificate requirement who have contraindications to live vaccines may be given an exemption certificate. However, they need to understand that if the disease is endemic at their destination they will be at risk of infection.

Meningitis ACWY

The only other time a traveller may be required to produce a certificate of vaccination is in order to obtain a visa to visit Saudi Arabia for the Hajj or Umra pilgrimages. In this case they require Meningitis ACWY immunization. This vaccine can be given by deep subcutaneous injection to individuals over 2 years old and confers 3 years' protection in 2–5 year olds, and 5 years' protection in those over this age. There is no official certificate for this vaccine so the patient-held record may be used, or the information about the vaccine (including date and vaccine given) simply written on practice headed notepaper and authenticated with a practice stamp. Meningitis ACWY vaccine can be given to individuals who have received the Men C vaccine, as long as at least 2 weeks have elapsed.

CONCLUSION

Offering travel health advice is about a lot more than vaccinations. It is important that the nurse recognizes all aspects of the subject and encourages the traveller to think about lifestyle issues in addition to vaccination.

Malaria risk has not been covered in this chapter, but the information sources given will introduce the nurse to this topic (see Further Reading). Travellers should be referred to an additional source of advice if the nurse does not feel confident to do this.

It is important to encourage the traveller to take personal responsibility for their health while travelling. The patient should be provided with a patient-held record of vaccination and be advised to present this whenever they seek travel advice.

ESSENTIAL SKILLS
• Perform a risk assessment
• Know where to obtain up-to-date information
• Offer individualized travel information and advice
• Administer appropriate vaccines

REFERENCES

1. Cossar J, Reid D, Fallon R, et al. A cumulative review of studies on travellers, their experience of illness and the implications of these findings. J Infect 1990; 21: 27–42.
2. Lea G, Leese J (eds). Health Information for Overseas Travel. London: HMSO, 2001. Available at: http://www.the-stationery-office.co.uk
3. Widerstrom L. Excellent booster response 4–6 years after a single primary dose of Inactivated Hepatitis A vaccine. Scand J Infect Dis 2002; 34(2): 110.
4. PHLS. Food and waterborne diseases associated with travel. CDR Weekly 12(27).
5. Department of Health. Immunisation Against Infectious Disease. London: HMSO, 1996.

FURTHER READING

Chiodini J, Boyne L. Atlas of Travel Medicine and Health. London: BC Decker, 2003.

Kassianos GC. Immunisation: Childhood and Travel Health, 4th edn. London: Blackwell Scientific, 2001.

Lea G, Leese J (eds). Health Information for Overseas Travel [Yellow Book]. London: HMSO, 2001. Available at: http://www.the-stationery-office.co.uk

Salisbury D, Begg N (eds). Immunisation Against Infectious Disease [Green Book]. London: HMSO, 1996. Available at: http://www.dh.gov.uk

WHO. International Travel and Health. London: HMSO, 2002. Available at: http://www.whoint/ith

USEFUL WEBSITES

Fit for Travel is a public-access site run by TRAVAX. It is an excellent site to recommend to patients: http://www.fitfortravel.scot.nhs.uk

TRAVAX online database is free to general practices in Scotland with a £50 per annum fee outside Scotland. However, members of the British Travel Health Association can access it free of charge. Telephone 0141 300 1132 for further information. http://www.travax.scot.nhs.uk

MASTA (Medical Advisory Service to Travellers Abroad) maintains its own site that general practices can subscribe to. Telephone 0113 238 7530 for further information. Public access site: http://www.masta.org

Chapter 3

Travel vaccinations that are sometimes recommended

Carolyn Driver

This chapter follows on from Chapter 2, which should be referred to for information on the importance of risk assessment and use of information sources when advising potential travellers. This chapter will look at those vaccines which fall into the 'sometimes recommended' category.

It is often the lifestyle that travellers adopt in their destination, rather than the destination itself, that is the most important factor in deciding whether these vaccines are required. The risk assessment component of the consultation is therefore vitally important.

HEPATITIS B

Hepatitis B (formerly known as serum hepatitis) is the second most common vaccine-preventable disease amongst travellers.[1] The infection is caused by the blood-borne hepatitis B virus (HBV).

An estimated 2 billion individuals have been infected and there are about 350 million chronic carriers of the virus worldwide. Carriers have a high risk of developing either cirrhosis or carcinoma of the liver. Hepatitis B is surpassed only by tobacco as a cause of cancer.[2]

HBV is transmitted in the same way as the human immunodeficiency virus (HIV) – by contact with blood or body fluids of an infected person. The main difference between the two infections is that HBV is 100 times more infectious than HIV. HBV has been known to remain infectious on environmental surfaces for at least a month at room temperature and only 0.00004 ml is required to transmit infection.[3, 4]

The world is divided into areas of low, intermediate and high prevalence of hepatitis B, and travellers from areas of low endemicity can grossly underestimate their risk when travelling to areas of high prevalence.

Travellers can put themselves at risk of HBV infection through unprotected sexual contact, tattooing, body piercing, acupuncture, or sharing razors, toothbrushes, or intravenous needles. Trauma is the most significant cause of morbidity in travellers and thus they may require medical treatment in areas where instruments are not adequately sterilized or where blood is not screened. Dental treatment is another potential source of infection in developing countries.

The risk of infection is more significant for those who travel to high-risk destinations for longer periods and for travellers indulging in risk-taking behaviour. Travellers should be counselled about the mode of infection for hepatitis B and informed of the availability of a safe, effective vaccine.

There are two licensed hepatitis B vaccines available in the UK plus a combined hepatitis A and B vaccine. The vaccines are inactivated and can be used from birth (except Twinrix because this contains hepatitis A which is licensed only for those aged 1 year and over). The vaccines should be administered intramuscularly into the deltoid muscle or, in infants under 1 year old, into the anterolateral aspect of the thigh.

Table 3.1 shows the different schedules that can be used, but bear in mind that spreading the three doses over 6 months is still the preferred regimen and should be used wherever time permits.

As both vaccines confer immunity in 96% of recipients who have completed a course, it is unnecessary to check for seroconversion and boosters are not required.[5] Advise patients that a blood test to confirm seroconversion can be

TABLE 3.1 Hepatitis B vaccination schedules	
Brand	Schedule
Engerix B paediatric (birth to 16 years)	0, 1, 6 months
	0, 1, 2 months plus a booster at 12 months
Engerix B adult	0, 1, 6 months
	0, 1, 2 months plus booster at 12 months
	0, 7, 21 days plus booster at 12 months
Engerix B adult May be used in children aged 10–16 years if they are unlikely to attend for final booster	0, 1 month (Confers long-lasting immunity, but if the patient does present at 6 months they can be given the paediatric product as a booster)
Twinrix	0, 1, 6 months *or*
	0, 7, 21 days plus booster at 12 months (This accelerated regimen is not licensed for Twinrix paediatric)
HBVAXPRO 5 µg (birth to 16 years)	0, 1, 6 months
	0, 1, 2 months with booster at 12 months
HBVAXPRO 10 µg (adults)	0, 1, 6 months
	0, 1, 2 months with booster at 12 months

performed at least 8 weeks after completion of a primary course if the individual wishes.

RABIES

Rabies is caused by a lyssavirus, which occurs primarily in animals and leads to an acute encephalomyelitis that is fatal once symptoms are present. The average incubation period is 3–8 weeks, but can be anywhere between 9 days and 6 years. Rabies causes an acute febrile illness with rapidly progressive central nervous system symptoms, which can include agoraphobia, agitation, aversion to mirrors, hydrophobia, hallucinations, dysphagia, convulsions and, ultimately, paralysis.

Worldwide there are an estimated 40,000–70,000 human deaths from rabies each year.[6] The virus may be carried by any carnivorous animal, but dogs and cats (and occasionally bats) are the most likely to transmit the virus to humans. Rabies is present in all continents except Australasia and Antarctica. Developed countries have managed a high degree of control so that the reservoir is primarily in the wild animal population, but in developing countries the dog is responsible for most human rabies deaths.

As it is impossible to anticipate whether or not a traveller will encounter a rabid animal, prevention measures should be taught to all (Box 3.1).

Post-exposure rabies treatment is very successful if started promptly, but travellers who will be remote from major cities or who will be travelling to developing countries where good post-exposure treatment (including rabies-specific immunoglobulin) may not be available should consider pre-exposure vaccination. This ensures that there are circulating antibodies already in the individual's system. Because of the extremely severe consequences of infection with rabies it is always advisable to seek post-exposure boosters after a bite. If, however, it takes some time to reach medical care there will be an immediate booster response, leading to high levels of circulating antibodies and rabies immunoglobulin will not be necessary.

In the UK two types of rabies vaccine are available. Both are modern cell-cultured vaccines:

- Human diploid cell vaccine (HDCV; Aventis Pasteur MSD). Licensed schedule: three-dose regimen, 1 ml given intramuscularly in the deltoid on days 0, 7 and 28. Booster recommended for those at high continuing risk 2–3 years later.
- Purified chick embryo cell vaccine (Rabipur; Chiron; distributed in the UK by MASTA). Licensed schedule: three-dose regimen, 1 ml given intramuscularly as above, on days 0, 7 and 21 or 28. Booster recommended for those at continued risk 2–5 years later.

Both vaccines can be given from birth and contra-indications to pre-exposure vaccine are as for all

---

BOX 3.1   Rabies prevention

- **Avoid contact with animals** especially dogs, cats, monkeys – parents need to ensure their children understand the importance of this.
- **Commence post–exposure vaccination as soon as possible.** This should consist of an injection of rabies-specific immunoglobulin (half infiltrated around the wound and the remainder given intramuscularly) and commencement of a course of modern cell-cultured rabies vaccination. (*Note*: It is never too late to start post-exposure treatment should a patient present weeks or months after a potential exposure).
- **If a bite or scratch does occur** wounds should be washed thoroughly under running water or any safe liquid and kept clean and dry while medical attention is sought.

inactivated vaccines. Side-effects are also similar and this is a generally well-tolerated vaccination.

Note: there is evidence that 0.1 ml of vaccine given intradermally using the same regimen confers good immunity. However, this schedule is unlicensed in the UK and a nurse should only administer it by this route with the authorization of his or her employer and if he or she is trained in intradermal injection technique. The advantage to the traveller of this route is that it is cheaper, because one ampoule of vaccine can be split between several recipients.

JAPANESE ENCEPHALITIS

Japanese encephalitis is caused by a flavivirus, which is transmitted to man by the Culex mosquito. The disease is endemic throughout south-east Asia.

Endemic areas

Domestic pigs and wading birds are reservoirs for the virus and rural farming areas are of greatest risk. Various studies have tried to estimate risk of transmission to tourists. There are two factors that make the risk assessment different from that for other insect-borne infections:

- Unlike the anopheline mosquito (responsible for transmitting malaria), which feeds exclusively on humans, the Culex feeds on various animal and bird hosts as well as humans. This reduces the odds of infected mosquitoes feeding on humans.
- The disease does not amplify in the infected human. Domestic pigs and wading birds are the only two species that amplify the infection (i.e. mosquitoes must bite these species to become infected).

It has been estimated that even in hyperendemic areas the infection rate among mosquitoes does not exceed 3% and the Center for Disease Control in Atlanta, USA, has estimated that the overall risk of Japanese encephalitis for short-term travellers is as low as 1 in 1 million.[7]

The travellers who are most likely to be at risk are those travelling to rural parts of south-east Asia for long periods or those who will be living and working in an agricultural setting. Risk is highest during or just after the rainy season, when mosquitoes are breeding, and this also needs to be considered in the risk assessment.

Prevention relies on mosquito-bite avoidance and for those at significant risk there are two unlicensed vaccines available in the UK, which

TABLE 3.2 Japanese encephalitis vaccine schedules		
Brand	**Schedule**	**Duration of protection**
JEVaccine (Biken) (Aventis Pasteur)	0, 7, 28 days	2 to 3 years
	1 ml by subcutaneous injection	
	0.5 ml for children aged 1–3 years	
Korean Green Cross (MASTA)	0, 7–14 days	1 year
	1 ml by subcutaneous injection	
	0.5 ml for children aged 1–3 years	
	0, 1, 2 months plus booster at 12 months	
	0, 7, 21 days plus booster at 12 months	

can be given on a named-patient basis (Table 3.2). These cannot be given under a patient group direction, but GPs can write individual private prescriptions.

Contraindications are as for any inactivated vaccine, but atopic individuals and those who have severe reactions to insect bites have a higher incidence of allergic reactions to this vaccine.[8] Allergic reactions following vaccination with Japanese encephalitis vaccine can be delayed and it is recommended that the course is completed at least 10 days prior to departure from the UK so that appropriate treatment would be available should this occur.

TICK-BORNE ENCEPHALITIS

Tick-borne encephalitis is caused by a flavivirus and occurs in parts of Scandinavia, central and eastern Europe and the western part of the former USSR. Transmission mainly occurs from April to August, but may extend outside these months in unseasonably warm weather.

Those most at risk are individuals working or camping in forests or those on walking holidays which involve considerable time spent in wooded areas. The ticks that transmit the virus brush off animals in the undergrowth and can then attach themselves to anything that subsequently brushes against the foliage.

Prevention involves appropriate protection via clothing and insect repellents. An unlicensed vaccine (Encepur) is available in the UK for those at significant risk and can be ordered on a named-patient basis from MASTA. The schedule most commonly used for travellers is two doses given intramuscularly 4 weeks apart, and a booster can be given at 12 months for those at continued risk.[9]

All those visiting endemic areas should be encouraged to inspect themselves for ticks after venturing into wooded areas. Medical advice should be sought if a tick is discovered and immunoglobulin may be available for post-exposure use.

SUMMARY

As none of the vaccines discussed in this chapter are compulsory their use is determined by thorough risk assessment and discussion with the traveller to enable him or her to make an informed decision about which vaccines they wish to receive.

The travel health adviser should refer to other resources and must always check if there will be a malaria risk at the destination.

Unlicensed vaccines

The two unlicensed vaccines mentioned in this chapter are both licensed and widely used in many other parts of the world.

The vaccines have not been licensed in the UK because the small demand means it is not worth the producers going through the costly licensing procedures.

When an unlicensed product is used the responsibility lies with the prescribing doctor, who should only proceed if the patient has given informed consent after a careful discussion about relative risks and benefits.

Nurses who give unlicensed vaccines should ensure they have the correct guidelines approved by their employer and that individual private prescriptions are signed.

ESSENTIAL SKILLS

- Ability to perform a risk assessment
- Knowing where to obtain up-to-date information
- Ability to offer individualized travel information and advice
- Administration of appropriate vaccines (according to employer-approved guidelines and signed privateprescription for any unlicensed vaccines)

REFERENCES

1. Loscher T, Keystone J, Steffen R. Vaccination of travellers against hepatitis A and B. J Travel Med 1999; 6: 107–114.

2. WHO. Hepatitis B. Fact Sheet WHO/204. Revised October 2000. Available at: http://www.who.int/inf-fs/en/fact204.html

3. Atkinson W, Wolfe C, Humiston S, Nelson R. Epidemiology and Prevention of Vaccine-Preventable Diseases, 6th edn. Atlanta: Center for Disease Control, 2000.

4. Kassianos G. Immunisation: Childhood and Travel Health, 4th edn. London: Blackwell Scientific, 2001.

5. European Consensus Group on Hepatitis B Immunity. Are booster immunisations needed for lifelong hepatitis B immunity? Lancet 2000; 355: 561–565.

6. WHO. Rabies – Fact Sheet N99. June 2001. Available at: http://www.who.int/inf-fs/en/fact099.html

7. Center for Disease Control. Inactivated Japanese encephalitis virus vaccine: recommendations of the advisory committee on immunisation practices (ACIP). MMWR 1993; 42(RR-1): 6.

8. Plesner A, Ronne T, Wachmann H. Case–control study of allergic reactions to Japanese encephalitis vaccine. Vaccine 2000; 18: 1830–1836.

9. Lea G, Leese J (eds). Health Information for Overseas Travel. London: HMSO, 2001. Available at: http://www.the-stationery-office.co.uk/doh/hinfo/index.htm

USEFUL WEBSITES

Fit for Travel is a public-access site run by TRAVAX. It is an excellent site to recommend to patients: http://www.fitfortravel.scot.nhs.uk

TRAVAX online database is free to general practices in Scotland with a £50 per annum fee outside Scotland. However, members of the British Travel Health Association can access it free of charge. Telephone 0141 300 1132 for further information. http://www.travax.scot.nhs.uk

MASTA (Medical Advisory Service to Travellers Abroad) maintains its own site that general practices can subscribe to. Telephone 0113 238 7530 for further information. Public access site: http://www.masta.org

Chapter 4

Advice on malaria

Carolyn Driver

The travel health consultation is a time-consuming health promotion exercise, and one that is becoming more complicated as people travel further afield. For many destinations, malaria prevention is one of the most important issues to be discussed. There are several good information sources to help the nurse determine whether the traveller is likely to be at risk and to suggest which medications should be considered.

It is always important to encourage the use of bite-avoidance measures (Box 4.1) as well as discussing chemoprophylaxis (Table 4.1).

WHAT IS THE CAUSE?

Travellers are more likely to comply with the complex instructions for malaria prophylaxis if they have a basic understanding of what the disease is and why medications must be taken for the prescribed lengths of time.

Malaria is a potentially fatal infection caused by a microscopic parasite called *Plasmodium*, which is transmitted to humans by the mosquito and requires both hosts to complete its lifecycle. There are many species of *Plasmodium*, but only four that affect humans:

- *Plasmodium falciparum*
- *Plasmodium ovale*
- *Plasmodium vivax*
- *Plasmodium malariae*.

BOX 4.1   Bite-avoidance measures

Clothing
- Cover as much skin as possible to reduce the opportunities for insects to bite

Insect repellents
- Should contain diethylmethyltoluamide
- Apply to all exposed skin
- Use up to 50% solution on adult skin and 10–20% for infants and children[1]

Insecticides
- Can be sprayed into the surrounding environment
- Can be used on clothing (natural fibres only) or applied to cotton wrist and ankle bands

Mosquito nets
- Essential if sleeping accommodation is not air-conditioned
- Should be treated with an insecticide such as permethrin

Vaporizers
- Plug-in devices that heat a permethrin-soaked mat
- Coils that give off a pyrethroid vapour when lit

Knock-down fly sprays
- Use in sleeping accommodation, especially when there is no air-conditioning

TABLE 4.1   Chemoprophylaxis regimens

Drug	Dose	Schedule
Adults		
Mefloquine (Lariam)	250 mg weekly	Commencing 2 weeks before travel and continued until 4 weeks after leaving infected area
Doxycycline	100 mg daily	Commencing 3 days before travel and continued until 4 weeks after leaving infected area
Atovaquone/proguanil (Malarone)	One tablet daily	Commencing 1 day before travel and continued for 7 days after leaving infected area
Children		
Drug	Body weight	Schedule (start and finish times as per adult dose)
Malarone	11–20 kg	One paediatric tablet per day
	21–30 kg	Two paediatric tablets per day
	31–40 kg	Three paediatric tablets per day
	> 40 kg	One adult tablet per day

Doxycyline is not recommended for children. For information on children's doses for mefloquine see the BNF.[3]

P. falciparum is the most serious infection and can become life-threatening very quickly if left untreated.

Malaria is transmitted by the female anopheline mosquito. When she bites, she injects a small inoculum into the bloodstream. This contains an anticoagulant that enables her to feed (Figure 4.1).

If she is already infected the inoculum will also contain about 20–200 sporozoites (microscopic single-cell parasitic organisms) that rapidly find their way to hepatocytes in the liver, where they reproduce. Cyst-like structures, called schizonts, are formed within 5–7 days in *P. falciparum* infection and within 30 days with the other species. Each schizont contains up to 40,000 merozoites (cells produced asexually by division).

When the schizont matures, it ruptures, releasing the merozoites into the circulation where they invade the red blood cells (RBCs) and feed on their contents. Reproduction continues and the RBCs burst, releasing merozoites back into the circulation where they invade fresh RBCs.

Some merozoites develop into a sexual stage, forming gametocytes. When another female anopheline mosquito bites, the gametocytes are taken into her stomach where they become sporozoites. These accumulate in her salivary glands ready to be injected into a new human host during her next meal. Thus the cycle is completed.[2]

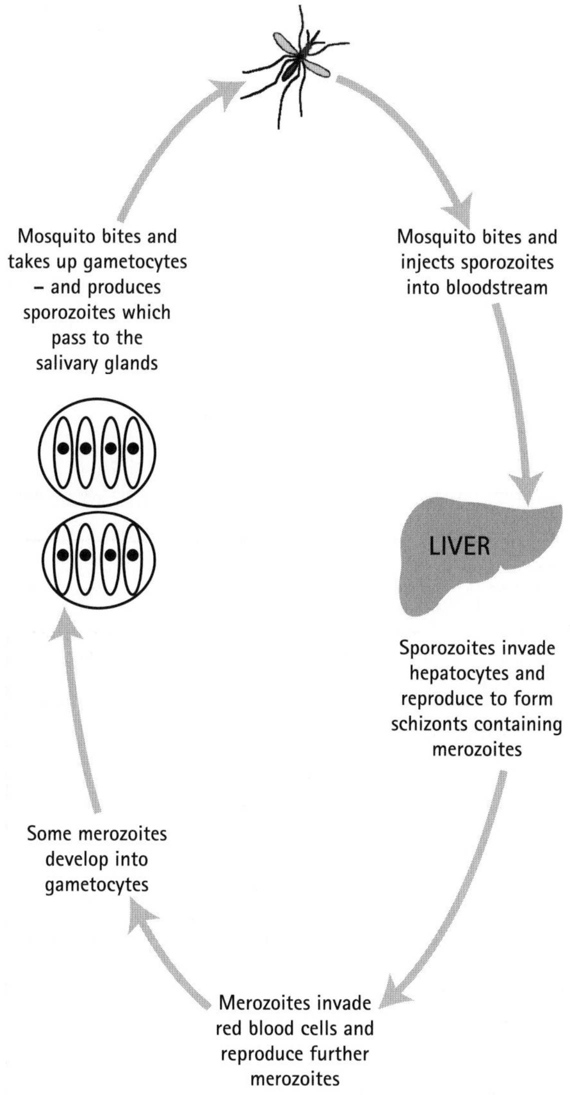

Mosquito bites and takes up gametocytes – and produces sporozoites which pass to the salivary glands

Mosquito bites and injects sporozoites into bloodstream

LIVER

Sporozoites invade hepatocytes and reproduce to form schizonts containing merozoites

Some merozoites develop into gametocytes

Merozoites invade red blood cells and reproduce further merozoites

Figure 4.1   Lifecycle of *Plasmodium*.

PREVENTION

Malaria prevention requires an understanding of how the disease is transmitted and an awareness of the combination of methods needed to avoid infection. The nurse can use an ABCD guide to educate the traveller:

- **A**: awareness
- **B**: bite avoidance
- **C**: chemoprophylaxis
- **D**: diagnosis.

Travellers who follow this guidance must be made aware that they still face a risk of contracting malaria, so they need to be vigilant about reporting their travel history should they develop a severe febrile illness within 2 years of returning from an endemic area.

Chemoprophylaxis

Chemoprophylaxis requires taking medication not only before and during travel to a malaria risk area, but also, in most cases, for 4 weeks after leaving (see Table 4.1). This is because most agents do not act until the blood phase of the disease. Compliance with such a regimen relies on the individual understanding the nature of the risk and the action of the drug.

Bite avoidance

None of the antimalarial drugs currently available offers 100% protection, so it is important for travellers to try to avoid being bitten by mosquitoes. Bite avoidance also prevents the spread of other insect-borne diseases, many of which cannot be prevented by vaccination or chemoprophylaxis.

Travellers need to know the various precautions to take (see Box 4.1).

CHOICE OF ANTIMALARIAL DRUG

The side-effects of currently available chemoprophylaxis agents range from minor gastric upset to neuropsychiatric symptoms (an emotive term encompassing headache, insomnia and dizziness), through to major psychotic episodes. Symptoms at the milder end of the spectrum are by far the more common, and can occur just as readily with chloroquine and proguanil as with mefloquine.[4]

Making the correct choice of antimalarial drug requires a balancing act between personal medical history, disease resistance and the degree of risk. In all cases an up-to-date *British National Formulary* should be used to check dosages, interactions and possible side-effects before prescribing.[4] The patient can then be advised about the different types of chemoprophylaxis that are suitable, and allowed to make an informed choice. Typical regimens are summarized in Table 4.1.

The medications require a private prescription from the GP, and the traveller then purchases the tablets from a pharmacist at the retail price. Many of the drugs are expensive, and can mean a significant cost for large family groups. However, travellers who have been correctly advised should understand that it is vital to buy the correct medication for themselves and their families.

Cost must not obstruct the decision-making process. However, the travel health adviser has a responsibility to give appropriate advice based on good information sources, and to make sure drugs are recommended only when there is a risk and where alternatives are not appropriate.

Mefloquine

Mefloquine is highly effective during the blood phase of the *Plasmodium* lifecycle. It has a long half-life, and thus needs to be taken only once a week. However, resistance to mefloquine has been observed in the Thai/Cambodian and Thai/Myanmar borders and the situation is being carefully monitored.

Mefloquine can be used in children from the age of 3 months, and in the second and third trimesters of pregnancy. Pregnancy should be avoided for 3 months after completing a course of the drug.

A history of depression, other mental health disorder or epilepsy in the individual or a first-degree relative are absolute contraindications to use of mefloquine. Caution is required if the patient has a cardiac conduction disorder or is taking beta blocker or calcium channel blocker drugs.

Doxycycline

Doxycycline is highly effective during the blood phase of the disease. It needs to be taken for just 2–3 days before entering an endemic area and then continued until 4 weeks after departure. Currently there is no evidence of resistance to doxycycline.

The drug cannot be used during pregnancy, lactation or in children under 12 years old. It is contraindicated in individuals with an allergy to tetracyclines.

Absorption is impaired by antacids containing aluminium, calcium or magnesium, and may also be reduced if taken concurrently with antiepileptic drugs.

Women using some oral contraceptive pills need to take additional precautions for the first 2 weeks of concurrent administration. Some women become more susceptible to candidal infection while taking doxycycline, so it is a wise precaution to pack a self-treatment preparation.

Photosensitivity is a potential adverse reaction to doxycycline, and may be reduced by observing sensible sun-protection precautions and using a high-factor sun screen (over 15) that blocks both ultraviolet A and B rays.[1, 5]

Atovaquone plus proguanil (Malarone)

Malarone destroys *P. falciparum* in both the liver and the blood phases of the disease. For this reason it needs to be taken for just 7 days after leaving an endemic area and it can be started 1 day before arrival, so patients have a considerably shorter course of medication. It is very well tolerated, comparing favourably with placebo during clinical trials. As with all antimalarial drugs, patients may experience headache and gastrointestinal disturbance.

The treatment is contraindicated in anyone with severe renal impairment or a known hypersensitivity to either component.

There are not yet enough data to support the use of Malarone in pregnancy. It is currently licensed for use for 1 day before arrival in the endemic area, up to 28 days while at risk, plus 7 days after (a maximum of 36 days).

A paediatric tablet is available and can be used for children weighing over 11 kg. Malarone is best taken with a meal. If a child is unable to swallow tablets the dose can be crushed into food, ideally strongly flavoured substances such as peanut butter or chocolate spread that mask the bitter taste. It is important to make sure the whole dose has been taken, so a very small quantity of the chosen food should be used.

Malarone is significantly more expensive than the alternatives, but the good side-effect profile and shorter course may outweigh this consideration in many cases.

Chloroquine and proguanil regimens

Chloroquine may be used for travel to the small number of destinations where resistance is not significant. For example, it can be used alone in Central America, or in combination with proguanil in the Indian subcontinent.

Chloroquine 300 mg/week is a cheap and effective regimen that has been in use for 50 years. It is contraindicated in anyone with a family history of epilepsy and in people with generalized psoriasis. It is safe to use during pregnancy.

Proguanil 200 mg/day is rarely used alone, although it is a possibility if chloroquine is contraindicated and the traveller will be visiting chloroquine-sensitive areas. It can be used in combination with weekly chloroquine when there is evidence of early chloroquine resistance.

There are no absolute contraindications to proguanil, but caution is advised in severe renal impairment. It is safe in pregnancy, but folate supplements are recommended.

It is generally recommended that chloroquine and proguanil are commenced 1 week before entering endemic areas, and both drugs must be continued for 4 weeks after leaving.

THE DIAGNOSIS

Patients show no sign of having acquired malaria until the disease starts to destroy the RBCs, usually 6–7 days after the initial infection. Indeed, malaria can usually be excluded if a patient develops symptoms less than a week after entering an endemic area.

Once the disease reaches the blood stage, patients may experience fever, chills, sweats, headaches, myalgia, nausea and vomiting, and occasionally cough.[4] These symptoms are similar to those of many viral infections, and thus the diagnosis is often missed or delayed. Travellers who are going to visit malarial areas must be warned to seek urgent medical attention if they develop a fever or flu-like illness.

Diagnosis can be made only by examining thick and thin blood films. A thick film screens a larger volume of blood and shows whether malaria infection is present. A thin film allows more microscopic examination and demonstrates the type of parasite and degree of parasitaemia (level of infection) present.[5]

P. falciparum can cause a rapid illness, resulting in multiple organ failure and death, sometimes within as little as 24 hours. Early diagnosis and treatment are vital to prevent such fatalities.[4] *P. ovale* and *P. vivax* may have greatly increased 'incubation' periods because they form hypnozoites, or dormant cells, in the liver phase of the infection. These may take months or even years to become active.

ADVICE FOR NURSES DEALING WITH TRAVELLERS

Nurses who advise travellers must understand the importance of establishing whether there is a malaria risk and have practice guidelines outlining how such consultations should be dealt with.

Most malaria chemoprophylactic drugs are prescription-only, and a nurse should be responsible for making recommendations only if he or she is competent to do so.

Although there is not, as yet, any national standard for training in travel health, there are several courses available (Box 4.2).

Nurses should always adhere to the Nursing and Midwifery Council guidelines and that means not engaging in any activity unless adequately trained to do so.

ESSENTIAL SKILLS

- Basic understanding of malaria
- Knowledge of resources to use to establish if traveller is at risk
- Knowledge of prevention methods so these can be discussed with traveller

---

BOX 4.2   Travel health courses

- **Diploma, MSc and Foundation Courses in Travel Medicine (Glasgow)**
  Contact: Travel Medicine Course Administrator, SCIEH, Clifton House, Clifton Place, Glasgow G3 7LN.
  Tel. 0141 300 1132. E-mail: TMdiploma@scieh.csa.scot.nhs.uk, or visit the TRAVAX website

- **Certificated Course (Lancaster)**
  Contact: Liz Hayward, Registry (Post-Professional), St. Martin's College, Bowerham Road,
  Lancaster LA1 3JD. Tel. 01524 384 384

- **Annual Residential Course (London)**
  Contact: The Registry, London School of Hygiene and Tropical Medicine, 50 Bedford Square,
  London WC1B 3DP. Tel. 020 7299 4648. Fax: 020 7323 0638. E-mail: shortcourses@lshtm.ac.uk.
  Website: http://www.lshtm.ac.uk

- **The Magister Course (Self-Directed Home Learning)**
  Contact: Richard Bazneh, The Old Rectory, St. Mary's Road, Stone, Dartford, Kent DA9 9AS.
  Tel. 01322 427 216

REFERENCES

1. Bradley D, Bannister B. Guidelines on prevention of malaria in travellers from the UK 2001. Communicable Dis Public Health 2001; 4(2): 84–101.
2. Warhurst D. The parasite. In: Schlagenhauf P (ed.). Traveller's Malaria. Ontario: BC Decker, 2001.
3. British Medical Association and The Royal Pharmaceutical Society of Great Britain. British National Formulary No. 51. London: BMA/RPSGB, 2006.
4. Barrett PJ, Emmins PD, Clarke PD, Bradley DJ. Comparison of adverse events associated with use of mefloquine and combination of chloroquine and proguanil as antimalarial prophylaxis: postal and telephone survey of travellers. BMJ 1996; 313: 525–528.
5. Beallor C, Kain KC. Doxycycline. In: Schlagenhauf P (ed.). Traveller's Malaria. Ontario: BC Decker, 2001.

FURTHER READING

Lea G, Leese J (eds). Health Information for Overseas Travel. London: TSO, 2001. Available at: http://www.the-stationery-office.co.uk/doh/hinfo/index.htm

World Health Organization. International Travel and Health. Geneva: WHO, 2003. Available at: http://www.who.int/ith and http://www.the-stationery-office.co.uk/doh/hinfo/index.htm

USEFUL WEBSITES

Advisory Committee on Malaria Prevention Guidelines. Comprehensive and regularly updated guidance for all healthcare professionals who advise travellers: http://www.malaria-reference.co.uk

Medical Advisory Service to Travellers Abroad. A public access site. Professional site also available on subscription; for further information call 0113 238 7530: http://www.masta.org

TRAVAX. Free to general practices in Scotland and members of the BTHA, and available for a yearly fee elsewhere: http://www.travax.scot.nhs.uk. A public-access site can be recommended to patients: http://www.fitfortravel.scot.nhs.uk

HELPLINES

Malaria Helpline. Tel. 020 7636 3924, Monday–Friday 9.00 a.m. to 4.30 p.m. For healthcare professionals.

National Travel Health Network and Centre. Tel. 020 7380 9234, 9 a.m. to 12 p.m.

Chapter 5

Injection technique, needle length and equipment

Kirsty Armstrong

There are many things to consider when performing vaccination for a child or an adult – whether as part of the national childhood immunization schedule or for travel. Many of these areas have been discussed in Chapters 1–3. This chapter deals with the importance of injection technique, needle length and correct sharps disposal.

A pre-vaccination checklist is given in Box 5.1, which you can copy and use as an *aide memoire* for those first few vaccinations that you have to do on your own, after you have had sufficient appropriate supervision.

NEEDLE LENGTH AND INJECTION SITE

If you give the vaccine incorrectly or with the wrong size needle you may cause damage to the patient and reduce the efficacy of the vaccine.[1]

Unless there are special circumstances, babies and infants should be given all vaccines (except the BCG) into the anterolateral aspect of the thigh (Figures 5.1 and 5.2). It is recommended that a 25 mm (1 inch) needle should be used to ensure the vaccine enters the muscle, where it will disseminate at the correct rate. Needle lengths and colours vary – some orange needles are 16 mm (5/8 inch) or 25 mm (1 inch) and 25 gauge, most blue needles are 25 mm (1 inch) length and 23 or 25 gauge.

BOX 5.1   Pre-vaccination checklist
✓ **Anaphylaxis pack** • Where is it and is your adrenalin up to date?
✓ **Check patient group directions** or protocols for this vaccine
✓ **Confirm patient details** • Especially for multiple family members especially twins
✓ **OK after previous vaccine like this?**
✓ **Any previous vaccine reactions?**
✓ **Any fever or contraindications?**
✓ **Immunocompromised** • Patient, family or co-habitees?
✓ **Any history of anaphylaxis/allergy/fainting?**
✓ **Obtain informed consent** • Give information on vaccine indications, side-effects, what to do in case of pyrexia and any other actions that parents/carers may have to take
✓ **Advise about efficacy, number of doses, boosters needed and schedules**
✓ **Check the drug** • Correct vaccine and package, expiry date, vial/syringe (for abnormalities). Note which vaccine, name and batch number, stage in course, site of injection and when next vaccination due in all relevant records
✓ **Check vaccine storage and reconstitution is correct and appropriate**
✓ **Prepare patient** • Make sure the treatment area is private, warm and safe, clean skin if necessary, use correct site and appropriate dose
✓ **Post-vaccination observation should be implemented if possible and appropriate** • Especially in atopic individuals, anaphylaxis is most likely in the first 20–30 minutes
✓ **Sharps disposal**
✓ **For travel vaccines should antibodies be checked?** • Advise patient what the vaccine will protect against (i.e. no vaccine is 100% effective), the live vaccine interval and when boosters are needed. Consider pregnancy.
✓ **Patient information leaflets**

Subcutaneous vaccines are the most irritating and using the 1 inch length needle will reduce irritation at the vaccine site and cause less pain. There are fewer pain receptor sites in muscles than in subcutaneous tissue.

Use prefilled syringes as supplied; if there is a choice of needle available use 16 mm (5/8 inch) for infants and 25 mm (1 inch) for older children. After the age of 3 years or in larger infants/children the deltoid can be used, but this is going to be most relevant in the administration of the pre-school booster (PSB). The needle should be inserted to the hub.

The PSB for the older child may be given in the deltoid aspect of the arm.[2] The intramuscular injection must be given at a 90° angle.

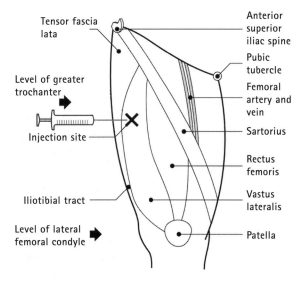

Figure 5.1 The muscles of the thigh and the recommended injection site.

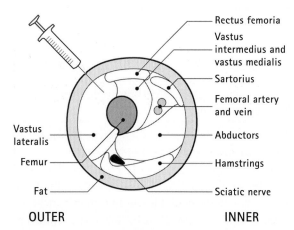

OUTER   INNER

Figure 5.2 Cross-section of the thigh showing the recommended injection site.

THE CUDDLE POSITION AND INJECTION TECHNIQUE

When administering vaccines to a baby, the child should be held firmly by the parent or carer, with the thigh exposed. The leg should also be held by the parent or carer – a member of staff may be useful here if the parent seems concerned about this.

Sterile swabs are no longer indicated before vaccination (wash with soap and water if very dirty), but a cotton wool ball is excellent for dusting off pre-vaccination and holding over the injection site post-immunization.[3]

After injecting the first site have the parent or carer hold the cotton ball and turn the baby round to expose the other thigh and inject that thigh in the same way. With older children I still suggest the child is on the lap of the parent or carer and I give a 'well done' sticker or maybe a sweet afterwards. Building bridges with children whom you may need to examine again in the future is vital.

A child's anxiety can be eased by a willing parent or carer who has primed the child – be wary of the parent who has not discussed the vaccination with the child.[2] It is worthwhile remembering that babies rarely faint but can often be shocked and pale after vaccination.

Adults with a needle phobia or who have not eaten recently are more likely to faint.[2] Inquire first and lie them down if necessary.

SHARPS DISPOSAL

Care is needed in sharps disposal. When you have a plethora of vaccinations to give use a clean kidney dish or disposable flat tray to hold all your vaccines together. This enables you to transport them safely, before and after immunization.

Many sharps injuries occur when uncovered needles are left on desks after immunization. This is less likely to happen if your used needles (which you *never* re-sheath) are in a walled tray.[4] You should identify the process you would go through in the case of sharps injury before you are in that situation.

A protocol, drawn up with all of your colleagues, of what you might do in an emergency is vital and will reduce stress in a crisis. Trays also help in the recording of the vaccines post-immunization, particularly when you have many babies to see and you may be using different batches and boxes. Record the vaccines and vaccine sites carefully on the record held by the parent or carer and the community health and medical records (paper or computer).

If you decide the child is not well enough to receive a vaccine, record the reasons. You may wish to check your decision with a colleague. You also need to identify when to review the child for the administration of the vaccine, as they will be unprotected until then.

Only draw up vaccines once you have the well and willing patient with you. Always discard unused drawn-up vaccines at the end of the session.

LOCAL AND GENERAL REACTIONS

One of the absolute contraindications to administering an immunization is a previous severe general reaction to the vaccine. Severe reactions would include:

- anaphylaxis
- prolonged unresponsiveness
- fever > 39.5°C within 48 hours of the vaccine
- prolonged inconsolable or high-pitched screaming for > 4 hours
- bronchospasm or laryngeal edema
- convulsions or encephalopathy occurring within 72 hours of the vaccine
- generalized collapse.

Local reactions are various and include slight swelling at the site (e.g. the size of a 50 pence coin) or redness around the injection site immediately after. More severe local reactions are indicated by an area of redness and swelling that becomes indurated (like orange peel) and involves most of the anterolateral aspect of the thigh or a major part of the circumference of the upper arm. The parent or carer should be warned about possible local reactions.

ORGANIZATION

Be organized and have everything to hand that you need. Poor organization and technique can endanger you as well as the patient. Make sure that you have appointments that are long enough to accommodate the injection, give the necessary information and complete the paperwork involved.

Never be afraid to ask for advice from a more experienced colleague, but remember that even someone who has many years of vaccination experience may not follow best practice. If in doubt do not vaccinate – mistakes made in haste are hard to rectify later. Children and babies will not judge you, but their parents will.

ESSENTIAL SKILLS

- Understand the different intramuscular injection sites for infants, children and adults
- Use appropriate needle size for each injection
- Use the 'cuddle position' for infants and young children
- Ensure excellent organization and technique
- Ensure safe sharps disposal

REFERENCES

1. Zuckermann JN. The importance of injecting vaccines into muscle. BMJ 2000; 321: 931–933.
2. Vaccine Administration Taskforce. UK Guidance on Best Practice in Vaccine Administration. London: Shire Hall, 2001.
3. Little K. Skin preparation for intramuscular injections. NT Plus 2000; 96(46): 608.
4. US Department of Labor. Occupational exposure to bloodborne pathogens; needlestick and other sharps injuries. Available at: http://www.osha.gov/SLTC/bloodbornepathogens/index.html

Chapter 6

Injections and immunizations

Kirsty Armstrong

This chapter examines some of the more unusual injections you may have to administer as a new practice nurse, as well as looking briefly at influenza and pneumococcal vaccinations.

If you are faced with an unfamiliar procedure or drug, or are in any doubt, consult with a more experienced colleague or your GP.

TRAINING AND COMPETENCY ISSUES

A pre-vaccination checklist is given in Box 6.1. In addition to the items listed there, there are some other issues that need to be addressed:

- If you are unfamiliar with a depot injection or technique do not administer it without first accessing appropriate training. Check with your local primary care trust (PCT) training and development coordinator about courses on offer.
- Many practices/PCTs do not use patient group directions (PGDs) – sometimes an up-to-date protocol will suffice until your PCT has produced these. If in doubt contact your PCT and check your legal standing.
- For products that are unfamiliar to you always check the *British National Formulary* (BNF), the special product characteristics (SPC) sheet and/or the data sheet supplied with the drug.
- Reimbursement of monies for vaccinations and medicines and the replenishment of stocks/

supplies tends to vary between practices. Your practice manager should work out the details, but you should keep careful records to provide all the information that is necessary.

BOX 6.1   Pre-vaccination checklist

✓	**Anaphylaxis pack** • Where is it and is your adrenalin up to date? • Check patient group directions or protocols for this vaccine
✓	**Confirm patient details** – especially for multiple family members (e.g. twins) • OK after previous vaccine like this? • Any previous vaccine reactions? • Any fever or contraindications? • Immunocompromised patient, family, or co-habitees? • Any history of anaphylaxis/allergy/fainting? • Obtain informed consent
✓	**Give information on:** • Vaccine indications and side-effects • What to do in case of pyrexia and any other actions that parents/carers may have to take
✓	**Advise about:** • Efficacy, number of doses, boosters needed, and schedules
✓	**Check:** **(i) the drug –** • Correct vaccine and package, expiry date, vial/syringe (for abnormalities)? Note which vaccine, name and batch number, stage in course, site of injection, and when next vaccination due in all relevant records **(ii) vaccine storage and reconstitution –** • Check vaccine storage and reconstitution is correct and appropriate
✓	**Prepare patient** • Make sure the treatment area is private, warm, and safe • Clean skin if necessary • Use correct site and appropriate dose
✓	**Post-vaccination** • Post-vaccination observation should be implemented if possible and appropriate – especially in atopic individuals, anaphylaxis is most likely in the first 20–30 minutes • Sharps disposal • Patient information leaflets
✓	**For travel vaccines** • For travel vaccines, should antibodies be checked? • Advise patient what the vaccine will protect against (i.e. no vaccine is 100% effective), the live vaccine interval, and when boosters are needed • Consider pregnancy

VITAMIN B$_{12}$

Pernicious anaemia is one type of megaloblastic anaemia that can occur after an autoimmune gastritis. It happens when there is lack of intrinsic factor (the mucoprotein that binds vitamin B$_{12}$) in the gut.

The patient is unable to absorb vitamin B$_{12}$ from their diet and will present with all the usual symptoms of anaemia, such as shortness of breath, pallor and fatigue. Once pernicious anaemia has been established as the cause of these symptoms hydroxycobalamin (Cobalin Hor Neo-Cytamen) is usually prescribed. The dosage is 250–1,000 µg on alternate days for 2 weeks, followed by 250 µg weekly until blood count is normal. The maintenance dose is 1,000 µg every 2–3 months.

Cyanocobalamin is also prescribed for pernicious anaemia, but it is not retained in the body for as long as hydroxycobalamin and so the maintenance dose needed is more frequent (once a month).[1]

Injections need to be given intramuscularly into the deltoid, alternating sites (e.g. swapping between right and left). Some patients, particularly if very thin, may prefer administration into the buttocks (gluteal muscles), but do be aware of the proximity of the sciatic nerve and only use the upper, outer quadrant of the buttock.

Patients can bring these injections to you from the pharmacy after dispensing on an FP10 (community prescription). You can keep them in your locked cupboard, clearly labelled for that patient only.

Iron

Iron is now seldom given intramuscularly, mainly because it causes discomfort and has no proven superiority over oral iron, provided the latter is well tolerated and the patient takes the tablets. The iron sorbitol intramuscular preparation Jectofer was discontinued in the UK in February 2003. Other preparations are available for administration by slow intravenous injection or infusion.

DEPOT INJECTIONS

Zoladex (Goserelin)

Goserelin is a potent hormonal manipulator (gonadorelin or LHRH analogue) and as such can be used for breast and prostate cancer, endometriosis and presurgery reduction of fibroids or down-regulation of pituitary receptors prior to super-ovulation in assisted reproduction.

Goserelin is a prescription-only medicine. You will need a PGD to administer this – an up-to-date protocol may suffice temporarily.

This treatment is administered as a depot subcutaneous injection. This means that you insert a slow-release capsule under the skin using the large-bore needle provided. The drug will be released gradually either over 1 month (3.6 mg) or over 3 months (10.8 mg).

The depot is inserted into the anterior abdominal wall. If you wish you can use lignocaine or ethylchloride as a local anaesthetic, which will require further training and another PGD. As the anaesthetic can sting, many patients prefer to have the goserelin inserted without it – they feel that the anaesthetic hurts more than the depot injection.

You will need to be trained on the insertion of the depot. This could be by another colleague who is practised at this, at a specific study day, or by the drug company, which can provide videos and dummies.

After insertion of the depot your practice can be reimbursed, usually by an FP 10 cimmunity prescription. Check with your practice manager or local PCT for guidelines.

Side-effects and contraindications

Many patients suffer no side-effects at all, while others may have hot flushes and headaches (mostly women) and men may suffer loss of libido.

In women the side-effects mimic the menopause as the drug suppresses oestrogen levels. It can reduce bone density in both men and women over time.

Leuprorelin

Prostap (leuprorelin) is another depot GnRH analogue. It differs slightly from goserelin in terms of indication and licensing, but is inserted in much the same way.

Contraception

Contraceptive injections such as Depo-Provera and Noristerat (medroxyprogesterone acetate) need to be administered under a PGD. You must be trained in family planning and understand the indications and contraindications.

Remember not to rub the area into which you have administered the injection as this may speed the process of dissemination.

Always give the patient her recall date. It is also helpful to make this date clear on the patient's records so that other members of the team are able to remind the patient if requested.

Antipsychotic drugs

Other depot injections that you may be asked to administer are the antipsychotic medications such as Depixol (flupentixol), Modecate (fluphenazine), Haldol (haloperidol), Piportil (phinothiazine) and Clopixol (zuclopenthixol). All these medications must be given by slow intramuscular injection into the gluteal muscle. Again you should avoid rubbing the area after insertion. Your patient should have been titrated slowly onto these medications after reduction from oral medications and may present between 2- and 4-weekly.

You may be asked to take bloods from time to time to monitor serum levels of the drug (if this is in your remit) and you can take this opportunity to check how the patient is feeling. With any type of depot, recall is vital. Give recall dates to all your patients and record them on notes or somewhere else where reception staff can access them easily.

These drugs have a number of side-effects and the patient must have close psychiatric follow-up

and/or intervention from their managing health-care professional. Doses are according to the patient's management plan.

ADRENALIN

Atopy is on the increase, especially nut allergy which can cause anaphylaxis.[2] Many patients will need to know how to administer their life-saving adrenalin pens. Placebo pens are available from the relevant manufacturer, and also leaflets and training if you need them.

Remember that the pens have a short shelf-life and all patients should have two pens in case they need to administer a second dose of adrenalin. Injection is by the subcutaneous route at a 90° angle to the skin. It can be administered through clothes if necessary.

Take the opportunity to talk to the patient about anaphylaxis and put him or her in touch with the relevant societies, who are extremely helpful. It may be useful for you to know that even members of the public can administer adrenalin using these pens as a life-saving procedure without fear of litigation. You, however, may need to be trained in their administration.

POST-EXPOSURE PROPHYLAXIS – IMMUNOGLOBULINS

You may come across post-exposure prophylaxis in many forms.

Rabies

A patient who has been bitten by a rabid animal may present to you with a management plan – following assessment and referral from the Public Health Laboratory Service (PHLS). You may be asked to give either rabies immunoglobulin and/or a course of rabies vaccines.

Any patient who has been assessed as at risk should have had a management plan and all the relevant vaccines issued by the PHLS. If in doubt contact the healthcare professional who has formulated the plan. The disease has a 100% mortality rate and any possible exposure must be taken seriously.[3] Patients will need multiple visits over a short period of time.

Varicella

At-risk patients may need to be administered varicella immunoglobulin where:

- there is a good patient history showing definite exposure
- a blood test has shown no antibodies to varicella (this is very unusual).

Patients at risk from varicella/herpes zoster include pregnant women (in the first and second trimester and close to birth), the immunocompromised (either through disease or treatment) and neonates (although you will not be treating this patient group).

Varicella immunoglobulin is also available from the PHLS.

POST-SPLENECTOMY PATIENTS

Patients who have had their spleens removed, either following trauma or as an adjunct to therapy in chronic disease, will need the 23-valent pneumococcal vaccine.

They may need a booster sooner than the 5-year recommended period if antibody levels fall. They also require the *Haemophilus influenza* type B (Hib) vaccine and the conjugate meningococcal C vaccine, if they did not receive these as part of the UK national programmes.

In addition, they need an annual influenza vaccination and will need ACWY if they are travelling abroad. Check with your local public health department, the patient and their specialist

before administering these vaccinations, as he or she may have already had some of the vaccine before they left hospital.

IMMUNOCOMPROMISED PATIENTS

Those individuals with the human immunodeficiency virus (HIV) or immunosuppression caused by treatment or disease may have suboptimal or fatal responses to vaccines. Those on high-dose steroids (e.g. for rheumatoid arthritis) and transplant patients are also immunocompromised. All these patients need careful, specialist supervision and advice.

Commonly requested vaccinations are conjugate meningococcal C, Hib, hepatitis B, pneumococcal, influenza, and occasionally MMR (measles, mumps and rubella) if the CD_4 and T-lymphocyte count are not too low.

Be aware that occasionally you may not know if a patient is HIV positive. A discussion about the vaccines before obtaining informed consent is vital.

OCCUPATIONAL RISKS

Hepatitis B vaccinations should be offered free to all those at occupational risk, but practice policies vary so do check with your practice and PCT. Those at risk include healthcare workers (e.g. doctors, nurses and dentists), sewage workers, refuse collectors, fire officers and those working in prisons.

Some PCTs also advise hepatitis A vaccinations. There are many different schedules, some extremely rapid (0, 7, 21 days with a booster at 12 months) and some more conventional (0, 1 and 6 months with serum levels checked at 4–6 months). Check the BNF for details and be aware of the rapid schedules, as they may not be included in your PGD or protocol. You may also be asked to vaccinate other high-risk individuals such as sex workers and long-term prisoners.

Rabies vaccinations may be needed for laboratory workers and vets, so check your local policy and charging procedure.

INFLUENZA CLINICS AND THE PNEUMOCOCCAL VACCINE

From early October flu clinics have to be fitted into every practice nurse's workload. Delegate as much of your administration as possible to reception staff and your practice manager, and ensure you have adequate supplies of this vaccine and plenty of room for storage.

Your practice manager should draw up a list of patients and, depending on resources, many patients will be invited by post. If possible, ask reception staff to organize your clinics with time at the end for any updating of records. At-risk groups are listed in Box 6.2. You may save time and appointments by also giving the pneumo-coccal vaccine to flu-clinic attendees – ask your practice manager to generate a list of those eligible who have not yet had this vaccination (Box 6.3).

As well as being good practice, you can make extra income by vaccinating those at risk. The Government has, however, increased the target levels to 70%.[4]

BOX 6.2   Groups at risk from influenza

- Patients with:
  - chronic respiratory disease
  - chronic heart disease
  - asthma
  - diabetes and other endocrine disorders
  - chronic renal disease
  - immunosuppression from disease or treatment
- Post-splenectomy patients
- Nursing-home residents
- Those aged over 65 years

BOX 6.3   Groups at risk from pneumonia

- Those with:
  - sickle cell anaemia
  - renal disease or nephritic syndrome
  - chronic obstructive pulmonary disease (COPD)
  - diabetes
  - immunodeficiency or immunosuppression/ HIV
  - liver disease and cirrhosis
  - heart failure
  - coeliac disease
- People who have undergone splenectomy
- Those aged over 65 years*

*See http://www.prodigy.nhs.uk/guidance.asp?gt= Immunizations%20–%20pneumococcal

---

PATIENTS PRESENTING WITH MEDICATION

Never give patients injections or immunizations from vials, ampoules or bottles unless they are labelled, they do not need to be kept refrigerated and have been prescribed by a recognized doctor or nurse prescriber. This is a legal and profess-ional minefield, so the practice should agree on a policy of administration.

Check that items have been stored at the right temperature if, for example, you are asked to give an injection of a fertility drug that has been prescribed by another GP or doctor. Check all

---

ESSENTIAL SKILLS

- Ability to master different injection techniques
- Awareness and application of PGDs, protocols and policy
- Knowing when to ask for advice from colleagues

your information thoroughly and be aware that any unlabelled, unrefrigerated medicines (possibly brought from abroad) could be a liability for you and your practice.

REFERENCES

1. British National Formulary, No. 51, March 2006. Available at: http://www.bnf.org
2. Hill D, Heine R, Hosking C. Management of peanut and nut allergies. Lancet 2001; 9250(357): 87–89.
3. Kassionos G. Immunisation: Childhood and Travel Health, 4th edn. Oxford: Blackwell Science, 2001.
4. Warmington V, James C. Hitting the mark: achieving target influenza vaccination. Nurs Pract 2003; Autumn: 51–52.

FURTHER READING

Department of Health. 12 Key Points on Consent: the Law in England. London: DoH, 2001. Available at: http://www.dh.gov.uk/consent

Resuscitation Council. Anaphylactic Reactions: Treatment for Adults by First Medical Responders. London: Resuscitation Council, 2003. Available at: http://www.resus.org.uk/pages/anaupdat.htm

Salisbury D, Begg N (eds). Immunisation Against Infectious Disease [Green Book]. London: HMSO, 1996. Available at: http://www.greenbook.gov.uk

Cervical screening

Maggie Cooper

Cervical screening is a method of preventing cancer by detecting and treating abnormal cell changes in the cervix (neck of womb). These abnormal cell changes can be a precursor to cancer of the cervix and can occur many years before the disease develops.

The epithelial cells on the cervix are subjected to a number of potentially harmful external influences during a woman's life; the most significant risk factor is the human papilloma virus (HPV). If abnormalities are not detected and treated appropriately, they may lead to more serious disease in later life.

THE SMEAR TEST

In England and Wales the cervical smear test is the current method of accessing and obtaining the appropriate cells from the cervix. A doctor or trained nurse, using a vaginal speculum to obtain access to the area, inserts an extended tip, wooden (Aylesbury) spatula into the ectocervix at the external os. A 360° sweep is taken twice round the area; this removes the exfoliated cells, which are 'smeared' onto a slide and sent to the local cytology laboratory for analysis.

LIQUID BASED CYTOLOGY

Liquid based cytology (LBC) has been introduced into the NHS cervical screening programme and is being rolled out throughout the UK. LBC is a new method of cervical cell sample preparation.

Cells are collected in the usual way, but with a Cervex brush instead of an Aylesbury spatula. The cell sample is then placed directly into a preservative fluid by either breaking the head off the brush and immersing it in the fluid or by rinsing the brush in the solution.

In the laboratory the samples are processed, much extraneous material is removed and a thin layer preparation is made on a slide, which is then analysed in the normal way. Training will be given when local laboratories adopt the new method and it is expected that the rate of inadequate smear samples will plummet (Box 7.1).

INCIDENCE AND MORTALITY

Cervical cancer is both painful and degrading. Incontinence of both bladder and bowel are often the result of direct spread of disease throughout the pelvis. Cervical cancer is, however, less likely to spread via the bloodstream to distant organs.

The worldwide incidence of cervical cancer is second only to breast cancer. Approximately 80% of cases occur in women from developing countries, which do not usually have screening programmes.[1] In the UK cervical cancer is relatively uncommon and is the eleventh most common cause of cancer deaths in women.[2] There were about 2,424 new cases of invasive cervical cancer diagnosed in 2001, and the incidence is falling year on year.[3]

Deaths from cervical cancer occur mainly in women over the age of 35 years and are now falling by about 7% per year.[3] Cervical cancer will never be eradicated completely, but it is likely that both the number of cases and the number of deaths from the disease would have increased markedly if the cervical screening programme had not been implemented. Cervical cancer incidence among women aged 20–64 years is estimated to have fallen by 44.6% between 1988 and 2000 in England (based on age-standardized rates per 100,000).[2,3]

Deaths in this age group also fell from about 6.9 per 100,000 in 1988 to about 2.9 per 100,000 in 2002.[2,3] This demonstrates the effectiveness of the current screening programme (Box 7.1).

RISK FACTORS

The precise cause of cervical cancer is not known, but there are a number of possible risk factors that may contribute to the development of the disease:[2]

- women who have not had regular screening
- certain strains of HPV have been detected in over 99% of cases of cervical cancer[2]
- women who have had (or whose partners have had) many sexual partners are at increased risk
- long-term use of the oral contraceptive pill could be a risk – the lack of barrier contraception playing a greater role than the action of the contraceptive pill
- women who smoke are twice as likely to develop the disease as non-smokers; mild abnormalities may regress if women stop smoking

---

BOX 7.1 Cervical cancer screening statistics for England, 2002–2003[3]

- 81.2% of women had been screened at least once in the previous 5 years
- 3.7 million women were screened
- 92.4% of the results obtained were negative
- 9.4% were inadequate samples (the smear cannot be interpreted – it may be too thick or too thin, obscured by inflammatory cells, blood, incorrectly labelled or does not contain the right type of cell)
- 3.9% showed borderline cell changes
- 2.2% showed mild cell changes
- 0.8% showed moderate cell changes
- 0.6% showed severe cell changes

- women who have pregnancies early in life and those who have many pregnancies
- women from lower socio-economic groups
- women who are immunosuppressed, either due to disease or to drugs, have less resistance to harmful viruses.

Many of these possible risk factors are behavioural rather than inherited, so women can exercise some control over them (e.g. by using condoms). Practice nurses can play a part in helping women to modify these risk factors by discussing this subject at routine consultations and by encouraging attendance for cervical screening.

SCREENING FOR CANCER

The purpose of screening for early detection of cancer is to interrupt the natural course of the disease and thereby prevent it from progressing to a more advanced stage and, ultimately, to death.[4]

What is a screening programme?

A screening programme is a set of activities with a common objective.[5] Cervical cytology is a screening tool that aims to detect pre-cancerous changes – not cervical cancer. Cervical smears are not diagnostic.

PRACTICE NURSES AND THE CERVICAL SCREENING PROGRAMME

Most cervical smears are taken in primary care, usually by practice nurses. Nurses who are working within the cervical screening programme should be prepared to advise, inform and educate women about the process. Cervical screening should not be viewed by employers as a simple, practical task such as taking blood or recording an electrocardiogram (ECG). Screening is a complex

process and, if not handled correctly, can cause as much harm as benefit.

The new practice nurse should not be expected to undertake this role until he or she has attended an accepted cervical cytology training programme, containing both theoretical and clinical components (see Recommended Training Courses at the end of this chapter).

It is important to know to which of your colleagues you may refer women for advice and information on cervical screening.

ANXIETIES AND MISCONCEPTIONS

Most women are anxious about having a smear test, for a number of reasons, including fear of pain and embarrassment. Inconvenience, lack of child-care facilities, expense and cultural inhibitions are also barriers that need to be overcome.

Well-person screening is poorly understood by the public. Some women believe that a smear test is a test for cancer and are consequently highly anxious about the test, the result and any possible follow-up.

As a new practice nurse you cannot be expected to be fully conversant with all aspects of the cervical screening programme, but by talking through the reasons for anxiety you can help to alleviate it.

WOMEN NEW TO THE UK

Women who enter the UK from abroad can pose some problems to primary care. Many countries do not have a cancer screening programme, and women may have no concept of health screening, compounded by language and cultural barriers. Other women may be used to having more frequent smears, taken by a gynaecologist rather than a nurse. The current policy is to invite women new to the UK for a smear test, once they have registered with a GP. This enables them to enter the UK system promptly.

WHO IS INVITED?

You need to find out the screening interval in your own area, how invitations and results are issued, and what leaflets are available for speakers of other languages.

Screening agencies invite all eligible women registered with a GP, using a computerized call and recall system.

New screening intervals were introduced in 2004 by the NHS Cervical Screening Programme and are now national policy in England and Wales:

- women will be called from age 25, not 20, but those aged under 25 years already in the screening programme will remain
- women aged 25–49 years will be screened every 3 years
- women aged 49–64 years will be screened every 5 years
- in Scotland the existing screening intervals of every 3 years for women aged 20–60 years will continue.

The first invitation is usually triggered on the woman's 25th birthday, but a woman can be invited at any time up to the age of 25 years. The woman is subsequently recalled according to the local screening interval.

The call/recall system also tracks any follow-up investigations that a woman might undergo and offers appropriate invitations, usually with a shorter time interval.

Computer systems in practice usually flag up defaulters from cervical screening and this is an opportunity for practice nurses, at other consultations, to issue a gentle reminder that the test is overdue.

WHO IS EXCLUDED?

- Women without a cervix (e.g. after total hysterectomy for benign reasons)
- women with terminal illness

- women who have never been sexually active are at very low risk of developing cervical cancer, but should make an informed decision whether they wish to be screened
- women who do not wish to take part in cervical screening are able to opt out, but need careful counselling about the risks and benefits of that decision.

RESULTS AND TREATMENT

All women should receive their results, in writing, within 6 weeks and most will receive a normal smear result. Women whose smear results show some degree of mild abnormality are usually followed up by increased cytological surveillance (more frequent smears).

Mild abnormalities often revert to normal without any intervention. Women with more severe cell changes are referred to colposcopy, where a gynaecologist using a low-powered microscope will examine the woman's cervix, in order to determine the severity of the problem and what treatment is needed. Colposcopy and treatment are usually carried out on an outpatient basis.

WHO IS INVOLVED IN THE CERVICAL SCREENING PROGRAMME?

GP practices

Practice nurses take most smear tests and GP practices need a robust system for ensuring that results are received for all smear tests taken. What happens in your surgery? Make sure you have copies of the recommended leaflets *Cervical Screening The Facts* and *Your Abnormal Smear*.

Family planning and sexual health clinics

Women have the right to choose where they have their smears taken and some choose to go to a

Family Planning or Sexual Health Clinic. Find out where these clinics are and the days and times that screening is offered.

Screening agency staff

The screening agency runs the computerized call and recall system, and sends invitations, reminder letters and results letters. Find out how long results take to come back in your area.

Cytology laboratories

Cytology laboratories interpret the smear tests. All slides are screened at least twice, and if abnormalities are found the slide can be screened up to four times. The cytology staff are made up of scientists and doctors. The cytology laboratory also passes the results on to the screening agency.

Colposcopy services

The colposcopy unit diagnoses the level of abnormality found in the cells and treats it accordingly. Patients are followed up and discharged back to primary care. Ensure you have supplies of the NHS leaflet *The Colposcopy Examination* and general information about your local colposcopy service.

Histology laboratory

The biopsy taken at colposcopy is passed to the histology laboratory, which reports back with a histological diagnosis.

Quality assurance

Regional quality assurance coordinating groups set and monitor standards for health authority activities, laboratories, colposcopy and primary care. They also identify training and research needs and offer advice.

THE IMPACT OF THE NHS CERVICAL SCREENING PROGRAMME

The UK Cervical Screening Programme is extremely successful. The UK screens more women than any other country and has the highest coverage. Screening is estimated to prevent 1,300 deaths per year.[2] Much of the fall in incidence and mortality of cervical cancer is attributable to the screening programme. Primary care plays a key role in this ongoing success, and practice nurses can feel justifiably proud of their contribution.

ESSENTIAL SKILLS

- Awareness of local expertise and available resources regarding cervical screening
- Knowledge of whom to refer women to for advice and information in your practice
- Familiarity with the basics of how the laboratory, call and recall agency, colposcopy clinic and primary care work together in cervical screening in your area
- Awareness of local screening intervals and recall arrangements
- Ability to convey a positive attitude towards screening

REFERENCES

1. Quinn M, Babb P, Jones J. Effect of screening on incidence of and mortality from cancer of cervix in England: evaluation based on routinely collected statistics. BMJ 1999; 318(7188): 904.

2. NHS. Cancer screening programmes: cervical cancer – incidence, mortality and risk factors. Available at: http://www.cancerscreening.nhs.uk/cervical/risks.html

3. Department of Health. Cervical screening programme,

England: 2002–2003. Available at: http://www.dh.gov.uk

4. Austoker J. Cancer prevention in primary care: setting the scene. BMJ 1994; 308(6941): 1415–1420.

5. NHS. Quality Assurance Guidelines for the Cervical Screening Programme. London: NHSCSP, 1996.

FURTHER READING

Austoker J. Cancer Prevention in Primary Care. London: BMJ Publications, 1995.

USEFUL WEBSITE

For a user friendly website with masses of information visit: http://www.cancerscreening.nhs.uk

RECOMMENDED TRAINING COURSES

The Royal College of Nursing offers some useful tips on where to access approved training for cervical screening. Visit their website at: http://www.rcn.org.uk. Courses include the following:

– Marie Curie Breast & Cervical Screening 4-day Course: accredited by Thames Valley University, 20 CATS points

– Marie Curie Cervical Screening Course: 2-day course

– Cervical cytology courses run in association with local laboratories, universities, QA teams and primary care organizations

– Developing Skills in Contraception and Reproductive Health Care: this course sometimes offers an additional cervical cytology module

Breast health

Victoria Harmer

This chapter highlights the importance of breast awareness and breast screening, and discusses the different benign breast conditions. Breast awareness is an effective and useful activity, and one that each nurse can promote and support.

THE ANATOMY OF THE BREAST

The breast is composed of fibrous, glandular and fatty tissue covered by skin. Fibrous bands divide the glandular tissue into approximately 15–20 lobes, and it is within these lobes that the milk-producing system can be found.

Each lobe contains up to 40 lobules that in turn contain 10–100 alveoli – the milk-secreting cells. The alveoli are connected to lactiferous duct, which is lined with epithelial cells. The alveoli are connected to lactiferous tubules; these lead to the lactiferous duct, which is lined with epithelial cells.

As it approaches the nipple, the lactiferous duct widens to form the ampulla, which acts as a reservoir for the milk to be stored. The lactiferous duct then continues on from the ampulla to open out onto the surface of the nipple.[1]

The glandular tissue of the breast is surrounded by fat. If weight is lost or gained, the breast will vary in size.

BREAST AWARENESS

Breast awareness is an important activity, and one that each woman can undertake. Breast awareness is based around the notion of 'getting to know your breasts' – how the breasts look and feel, and what is normal for the woman at different times of the month. If the woman notices anything unusual she should visit her GP immediately.

Although most women associate lumps in the breast or armpit with breast cancer, it is important to remember that nine out of ten lumps are not malignant. Women self-detect 75% of all breast cancers by checking their breasts, i.e. by being 'breast aware'.

Being breast aware is simple to do and does not entail following a strict or complicated routine. It just means women knowing what their breasts normally look and feel like, in any way that makes them feel most comfortable, for example in the bath or shower, when dressing, standing up or lying down. If anything unusual is found (Box 8.1), or a woman is worried, she should contact her GP as soon as possible because prompt detection and treatment of breast cancer offers the best chance of survival.

Although during pregnancy the breasts will change in size and texture, and possibly become tender, it is still important that the woman remains breast aware, reporting any worries to her GP or practice nurse.

Assisting women in becoming breast aware allows them to take more of an active part in their health, and can give them more control over their body. It is a simple yet effective part of health promotion, and one that nurses can easily endorse and facilitate.

Breast awareness leaflets are available from Breast Cancer Care or from local health authorities, and can be useful in teaching awareness to patients, as well as providing a useful guide for them to take home as a resource or memory aid.

COMMON BREAST DISORDERS

Breast disorders account for approximately 30 new patients per 1,000 women seen every year by a GP. In the UK, approximately 230,000 women with breast abnormalities are referred to hospital each year, with just under 6% of cases culminating in a diagnosis of breast cancer.[2]

Benign breast lumps should be referred to a specialist centre where triple assessment (clinical examination, radiological imaging and cytology/histology) can take place, in order to obtain a confident diagnosis. Criteria for referral to a breast care unit are shown in Box 8.2.

The main types of benign breast disorder are discussed below.

Mastalgia

Mastalgia can be divided into cyclical and non-cyclical breast pain, which is determined by using a pain diary to record when and where the pain occurs. Cyclical pain is experienced from mid-cycle onwards, and usually resolves on menstruation. This condition can last for years

---

> **BOX 8.1   Things to look for in breast awareness**
>
> Breast awareness should focus on:
>
> - any changes in the shape or size of either or both breasts
> - any change in either or both nipples – in appearance, direction or any blood-stained discharge
> - any dimpling or puckering in the skin of either or both breasts
> - skin changes – redness, dry skin, lumps
> - thickening in the breasts or axilla (in the armpits)
> - breast pain that does not go away after a period

BOX 8.2   Summary of conditions requiring referral to a breast care unit[3, 4]

Urgent referral (within 2 weeks)
- Patients 30 years old or over (the precise age criterion to be agreed by each network) with a discrete lump in the breast
- Patients with breast signs or symptoms that are highly suggestive of cancer. These include:
  - ulceration
  - skin nodule
  - skin distortion
  - nipple eczema
  - nipple retraction or distortion (< 3 months)
  - unilateral nipple discharge which stains clothes

Conditions that require referral, not necessarily urgent
- Breast lumps in the following patients, or of the following types:
  - discrete lump in a younger woman (< 30 years old)
  - asymmetrical nodularity that persists at a review after menstruation
  - abscess
  - persistently refilling or recurrent cyst
- Intractable pain that does not respond to simple measures such as wearing a well-fitting bra and using over-the-counter analgesics such as paracetamol
- Nipple discharge:
  - bilateral discharge sufficient to stain clothes in patients < 50 years old
  - bloodstained discharge in patients aged < 50 years (urgent referral required if discharge is unilateral)
  - any nipple discharge in patients > 50 years old

and, while it can vary in severity from cycle to cycle, it can affect activities of daily living.

While high-dose gamolenic acid (evening primrose oil) may be recommended, it can take up to 4 months before any benefit is noted. If unresolved, other drugs, such as danazol (Danol) or bromocriptine (Parlodel), may be prescribed, although these have an unwanted side-effect profile that includes facial hair, nausea and weight gain.

Non-cyclical breast pain affects older women, and may be random or continuous, localized in the chest wall or present as diffuse breast pain. It can be eased with the 24-hour use of a firm support bra and treated with non-steroidal anti-inflammatory drugs, or with those used for cyclical mastalgia, using gamolenic acid in the first instance.

Fibroadenoma

Fibroadenomas develop from a lobule in the breast, and make up 13% of all lumps in women aged under 20 years. There are four types of tumour: common, giant (more than 5 cm), juvenile and phyllode. Some disappear, one-third get smaller, and fewer than 10% increase in size. They can be left in the breast once diagnosed adequately through triple assessment, or surgically removed.

Cysts

Cysts are fluid-filled sacs that appear suddenly in one or both breasts and are often associated with pain. They feel like smooth, discrete lumps, and are more common in women aged 40–50 years old. Cysts can be aspirated to resolution, although if the aspirate is bloodstained a sample should be sent to cytology.

Duct ectasia

This presents either as a 'cheesy' nipple discharge, a hard or doughy breast mass, or by nipples that have retracted (become slit-like). It results from the retention of secretions after the age-related shortening and dilatation of milk ducts once they become redundant. Smoking increases the risk of duct ectasia.

Patients with duct ectasia may require surgical removal of the milk ducts (microdochectomy).

Epithelial hyperplasia

Epithelial hyperplasia develops from overgrowth in the lining of the terminal duct lobular unit, which results in general lumpiness, a lump or nipple discharge. The degree of hyperplasia can be graded as mild, moderate or florid.

If cytology shows atypical features, the condition is known as atypical ductal hyperplasia, and needs to be kept under surveillance as it can be a risk factor for breast cancer.

Duct papilloma

Duct papillomas are benign lesions of the milk duct or ducts, which result in single-duct nipple discharge. If discharge is prolific, treatment is by surgical excision; otherwise reassurance is sufficient.

Nipple discharge

This can be multi-duct or single duct, with the latter thought to be more indicative of breast cancer (5–8% is found to be ductal carcinoma *in situ*). Intraduct papillomas, duct ectasia and fibrocystic disease may also be the cause of discharge.

Lipoma

A lipoma is a common benign tumour composed of well-differentiated fat cells. It can be left with no clinical follow-up, or surgically removed for cosmetic reasons.

Mastitis/breast abscess

Mastitis commonly occurs from infection during breastfeeding, when bacteria enter through a cracked nipple and cause inflammation, causing the breast tissue to become hot, red and swollen. Antibiotics can relieve this, as can the use of a breast pump. In some cases an abscess may form, which will require multiple aspirations or surgical drainage.

If breastfeeding is not taking place, periductal inflammation may occur near the nipple area, and may progress to abscess formation. Sometimes the abscess will discharge itself and form a mammary fistula, which should be treated by a fistulotomy or fistulectomy.

Galactocele

A galactocele is a cyst that can occur during pregnancy or breastfeeding. It is caused by the blockage of a milk duct, probably due to inspissated (thickened) milk. This condition may resolve spontaneously or require aspiration.

Fat necrosis

Fat necrosis usually presents as an ill-defined lump resulting from trauma. It feels clinically suspicious, and looks worrying on a mammogram. Diagnosis through triple assessment is recommended.

Gynaecomastia

This is the enlargement of breast tissue in the male. It occurs in 30–60% of boys aged between 10 and 16 years, and 80% of cases will resolve spontaneously within 2 years. Surgical removal of the breast tissue is an option if the condition persists.

BREAST CANCER

The size of the problem

Each year there are approximately 10 million new cancer cases worldwide, with 10% arising from the breast, making it the second most common site of cancer after cancer of the lung.[5] In 2002, 22% of all new cancers in women were accountable to breast cancer, making it the most common site for cancer in women worldwide. In high-income countries the proportion of women with this disease rises to 27%, making it more than twice as common as any other cancer in females.[6]

Breast cancer in the UK

Of all cancers diagnosed in the UK, breast cancer is the most common female cancer, and accounts for 30% of all new cases. Each year in the UK over 40,000 cases of breast cancer are diagnosed and around 13,000 women die from the disease. The estimated lifetime risk for women is one in nine. Figure 8.1 shows breast cancer incidence in the UK according to age.[7]

Risk factors

The risk of breast cancer increases with a person's age. Other factors that increase the risk are: being female, late age at first pregnancy, low parity, early menarche and late menopause. The western world's lower population rates can partly explain the observed increase in breast cancer, and may predict an increasing incidence in areas where populations are declining.

NHS Breast Screening Programme

The Forrest report identified the criteria required to establish a screening programme,[8] and in 1988 the NHS Breast Screening Programme (NHSBSP) was set up in the UK, aiming to reduce mortality from breast cancer by 25% in the population screened. This national programme states that:

- women over 50 years of age should be invited for screening once every 3 years
- women attending should have one mammographic view of each breast taken
- the age range of women invited should be 50–70 years.

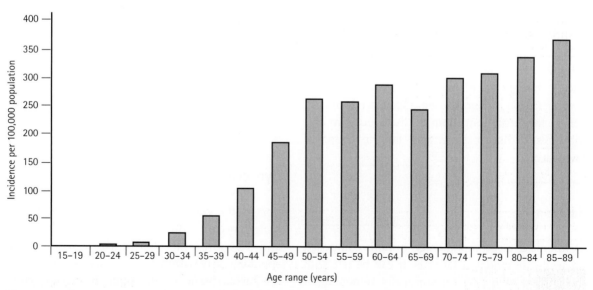

Figure 8.1   Breast cancer incidence in the UK according to age, 1995–1997.[7]

Women aged 70 years and over are entitled to, and can request, a routine screening appointment every 3 years, whether or not symptoms are apparent. The woman's GP can arrange this for her. Figure 8.2 illustrates the breast screening process.

Since the NHSBSP was established, over 15 million mammograms have been undertaken, and over 90,000 cancers have been detected. Between 1994 and 2004 in the UK, deaths from breast cancer in women aged under 70 years have fallen by 30%, with an estimated one-third of these attributed to breast screening. In the UK, the NHSBSP now screens approximately 1.5 million women annually. It is estimated that this programme will save 1,250 lives each year (25% reduction in mortality) by 2010.[9] In England, the budget for the breast screening programme is £52 million. Thus it costs about £30 per woman invited, or £40 per woman screened.[10]

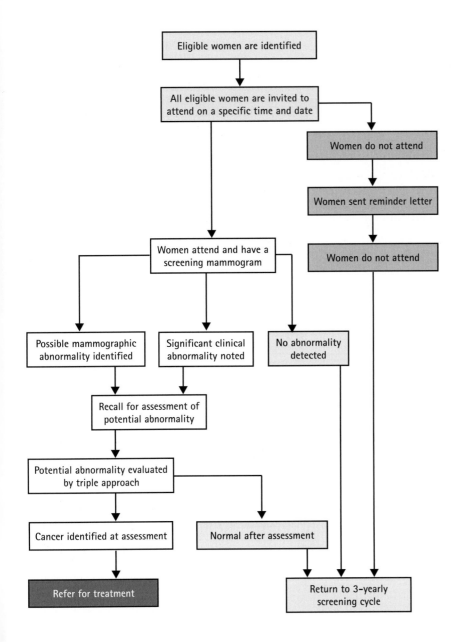

Figure 8.2 The breast screening process.

Natural history as related to screening

Survival after diagnosis and treatment of breast cancer is directly related to stage at diagnosis. The earlier the breast cancer is diagnosed the greater the treatment options, resulting in better survival rates. There is considerable potential for reducing mortality from breast cancer in populations by detecting breast cancer early. About 70–80% of cancers detected on screening may have a good prognosis. At the initial screen, up to 20% of cancers will be *in situ* with no ability to spread (almost a pre-cancerous stage), while those invasive cancers detected are small and less likely than larger tumours to have spread to local lymph nodes or metastasized to distant sites in the body.[11]

CONCLUSION

Breast awareness and breast screening are imperative for good breast health. An attempt has been made here to illustrate the salient points in this area, although it must be remembered that, if in doubt, referral to a specialist breast unit should be made.

Patients with benign breast disease need on-going support from healthcare professionals and continued awareness of any further changes to the breast. Each new lump found must be treated with a referral to a breast care unit to ensure an accurate diagnosis.

The nurse can act as an effective resource for people with breast problems, providing support and advice to improve the understanding of breast health and breast awareness.

ESSENTIAL SKILLS

- Knowledge of breast awareness
- An insight into benign breast disease
- An understanding of the NHSBSP and why it has proved a necessary and reliable programme in detection of breast cancers

---

REFERENCES

1. Grimsey E. An overview of breast cancer. In: Harmer V. Breast Cancer Nursing Care and Management. London: Whurr, 2003.
2. Leinster SJ, Gibbs TJ, Downey H. Shared Care for Breast Disease. Oxford: Isis Medical Media, 2000.
3. NICE. Guidance on cancer services. Improving outcomes in breast cancer. Manual update. 2002. Available at: http://www.nice.org.uk/page.aspx?o=36018
4. Department of Health. Referral Guidelines for Suspected Cancer. Available at: http://www.dh.gov.uk/PolicyAndGuidance/HealthAndSocialCareTopics/Cancer
5. Parkin DM. Global cancer statistics in the year 2000. Lancet Oncol 2001; 2: 533–543.
6. Vainio H, Bianchini F (eds). Breast Cancer Screening. IARC Handbooks of Cancer Prevention. Lyon: IARC Press, 2002.
7. Office for National Statistics. Breast cancer incidence according to age, 1995–1997. London: Office for National Statistics, 2001. Available at: http://www.statistics.gov.uk
8. Forrest APM. Breast Cancer Screening: Report to the Health Ministers of England, Wales, Scotland & Northern Ireland. London: HMSO, 1986.
9. Patnick J. Serving Women for 15 Years. NHS Breast Screening Programme Annual Review. Sheffield: NHSBSP, 2003.
10. Department of Health. NHS Cancer Screening Programmes. London: Department of Health, 2004. Available at: http://www.cancerscreening.nhs.uk/breastscreen/index.html
11. Austoker J. Cancer Prevention in Primary Care. London: BMJ Publishing Group, 1995.

FURTHER READING

Burnet K. Holistic Breast Care. London: Harcourt, 2001.

Harmer V. Breast Cancer Nursing Care and Management. London: Whurr, 2003.

USEFUL WEBSITES

Breakthrough Breast Cancer: Tel. 08080 100 200,
http://www.breakthrough.org.uk

Breast Cancer Care: Tel. 020 7384 2984,
http://www.breastcancercare.org.uk

Chapter 9

Contraception

Catriona Sutherland

Patients think of the practice nurse as a provider of nursing care and a source of information and advice on a broad range of illnesses and health promotion activities. Nurses who are new to general practice are likely to be asked questions on conditions and concerns that may not be within their field of competence. They then have to decide quickly whether they have the knowledge to provide an answer to the inquiry and, if not, where and how to make the most appropriate referral.

To meet patients' contraception needs, the nurse needs to know the basics, plus any information and services that can be provided in the practice, and who can provide them.

TRAINING ISSUES

Nurses who are new to primary care must comply with the Nursing and Midwifery Council (NMC) scope of practice guidelines. This means that advice on contraception can be provided only by those who have undergone appropriate training. Provision of emergency contraception may be an exception. This can be given by nurses who are not trained in family planning but who have received training on emergency contraception under a patient group direction. Essential skills for nurses offering advice on contraception are listed in the box at the end of this chapter.

THE CONTRACEPTION CONSULTATION

Contraception is a specialist area that needs dedicated skills. It is not solely about family planning. For some patients, access to contraception is the only reason why they contact the practice. Consequently, they use the contraceptive consultation as an opportunity to discuss other issues.

Because of the intimate nature of the contraception consultation, many women will also divulge or discuss their most private and sensitive concerns. Thus the nurse who handles the consultation is expected to be aware of a wide range of issues and be able to refer on as necessary. These concerns may include:

- sexual health
- sexual anxieties
- pregnancy planning
- unwanted pregnancy
- menstrual disorders
- fertility concerns
- sexuality
- cervical screening
- breast awareness
- domestic violence
- sexual assault/abuse.

BOX 9.1   Assessment of Fraser competency

- The girl (under 16 years old) will understand the advice given
- The doctor/nurse cannot persuade the girl to inform her parents or to allow the doctor or nurse to inform them that she is seeking emergency contraception and contraception advice
- The girl has or is likely to have had sexual intercourse with or without contraception advice/treatment
- That unless emergency contraception and/or contraceptive advice is given, her physical or mental health or both are likely to suffer
- That her best interests require the doctor/nurse to give emergency contraception advice without parental consent

---

Several methods are available in primary care:

- oral contraceptives
- emergency contraception
- injections and implants
- intrauterine devices and system
- barriers
- natural methods.

THE ESSENTIALS

The nurse needs to be well informed about the core issues in contraception, which include:

- confidentiality
- consent
- under-16 year olds and Fraser competency (Box 9.1)
- child protection.

The nurse also needs to have some awareness of the more commonly used methods of contraception, so the patient can be directed to the most appropriate person or place to meet her needs.

ORAL CONTRACEPTIVES

Combined oral contraceptives (COCs), such as Microgynon 30, Marvelon and Femodene, contain both an oestrogen and a progestogen. They are 99% effective if taken according to instructions. Their main mode of action is inhibition of ovulation, but they may also have an effect on sperm penetrability of the cervical mucus. The dose is fixed in most formulations, but in a few the dose is phased (usually with a higher dose in the latter part of the cycle). Most formulations are taken in a cycle of 3 weeks on followed by 1 week off.

Progestogen-only pills (POPs) such as Microval or Noriday are also 99% effective if used correctly. They act mainly by altering the cervical mucus to reduce sperm penetrability, but there may also be a considerable effect on ovulation, particularly in older women. Cerazette (desogestrel), a new POP, is actually designed to inhibit ovulation and has higher efficacy. POPs are taken daily without a break and may be taken where combined oral contraceptives are contraindicated (e.g. in migraine sufferers and when breastfeeding).

EMERGENCY CONTRACEPTION

Women who have had unprotected intercourse can obtain emergency contraception from any GP or from a trained family planning nurse. There are two methods:

- oral
- intrauterine.

Oral emergency contraception consists of two tablets. The first must be taken within 72 hours of the first or only episode of intercourse, and preferably within 24 hours; the second is taken 12–16 hours after the first. The efficacy is 95% if the treatment starts within 24 hours of intercourse, reducing to 85% after 25–48 hours, and 58% after 49–72 hours. Oral emergency contraception can be used more than once in one cycle. It is also available from some pharmacies at a cost of around £20–25.

The Royal College of Nursing is currently reviewing the guidance document advising practice nurses and others on the supply and administration of contraception under patient group directions (PGDs).

An alternative approach is to fit an intrauterine device (IUD) within 5 days of unprotected intercourse or up to 5 days after the earliest expected ovulation date (i.e. counting up to day 19 of a 28-day cycle). If a woman has an irregular cycle, the calculations are made on the shortest usual cycle.

INJECTIONS AND IMPLANTS

A long-acting injectable progestogen offers protection for 8–12 weeks. A subdermal progestogen implant, which must be fitted by a trained practitioner, is effective for 3 years, after which time the capsule has to be removed. Both methods are more than 99% effective, but periods are often irregular and some women experience acne, mood changes and tender breasts.

Intrauterine devices and system

Intrauterine contraception is fitted by a trained practitioner, but the practice nurse may be asked to assist, for example by sterilizing the equipment or caring for the patient.

Non-hormonal IUDs contain copper, and offer 98% to over 99% efficacy. They are long-acting, lasting 5–10 years, and low maintenance.

Mirena, the hormonal intrauterine system (IUS), releases a low level of progestogen. It lasts for 5 years and has beneficial effects on menorrhagia and dysmenorrhoea. Irregular light bleeding is common with the IUS for the first 3–6 months. Periods may become heavier, longer and more painful.

Barrier methods

If used according to the instructions, caps and diaphragms are 92–96% effective. A cap covers the cervix alone; a diaphragm covers the cervix and some of the vaginal wall. Neither the diaphragm nor the cap protects against the transmission of sexually transmitted infections through the vaginal wall.

Male and female condoms are 98% effective.

Natural methods

Natural birth control is based on predicting the time of ovulation, using indicators such as calendar, temperature and cervical mucus. If several indicators are used natural methods can be 98% effective. No hormones are used but the method involves avoiding intercourse at certain times and most people need guidance from a trained teacher.

New developments

There are two new combined oestrogen/progestogen methods: a transdermal patch and a vaginal ring.

The patch (Evra) is already available in the UK. Each patch is worn for a week, following a routine of 3 weeks on and 1 week off. One key advantage appears to be a high level of compliance among younger users.

The vaginal ring is available in the USA and in parts of Europe. It is used for 3 weeks, followed by a 1 week break.

The manufacturers of both these new methods claim that they are highly effective and well tolerated.

WHAT THE PRACTICE MAY OFFER

Most practices offer a range of oral and injectable contraception, and many can now provide a more comprehensive service, including the fitting of IUDs, the IUS, diaphragms and caps.

There are many initiatives around the country to make male condoms available, and some general practices now provide them with the support of the primary care trust.

Traditionally, GPs have received an item-of-service payment to provide contraception services. Under PMS (personal medical services) there are no longer individual fees, but instead there is an overall budget that reflects any enhanced service.

REFERRALS

If a patient's needs cannot be met in the practice, the GP can arrange a referral to a wide range of services (e.g. counsellor, continence adviser), some of which may be available on the same premises.

The practice nurse needs to be aware which services are available in the practice, nearby, or elsewhere in the area. Examples include:

- specialist contraception clinic (e.g. the local hospital trust may have a consultant clinic)
- sexual health clinic
- young people's clinic
- psychosexual counselling
- relationship counselling
- ultrasound scanning (e.g. for a 'lost' IUD)
- termination of pregnancy
- alcohol/drug services
- gynaecology
- colposcopy
- sterilization counselling.

PRACTICE SYSTEMS

Not every practice can provide every patient's chosen method of contraception. Some offer an extensive range, delivered by a large multidisciplinary team. Others have a much more limited service, or offer no contraception at all, perhaps for religious reasons. Whatever is available, the practice must have systems in place to ensure effective delivery. These systems will cover, for example:

- ordering and displaying the full range of current contraception leaflets
- ordering and displaying the full range of current sexual health leaflets
- advertising services available in the practice through the practice leaflet, posters, etc.
- pregnancy testing – this may be carried out by any member of the team but the result should be given by the clinician who requested it
- issuing condoms, ideally easily available from reception
- emergency contraception, ensuring ease of access for patients

TABLE 9.1   Hidden complexities in 'simple' requests

Request	Possible complexities
I only need some more pills	You do not know what pills the woman is taking, whether she is taking them correctly, or if she now has any contraindication to the COC or POP
I only need some more pills, but I am late starting back on them	People's idea of 'late' varies. The woman may be at risk of pregnancy, in need of emergency contraception, or already pregnant
I need my next injection. I don't know when I had my last one, but I must be due around now	Correct timing of injections is very important. The woman may be at risk of pregnancy, in need of emergency contraception, or already pregnant
I want to change to the pill my friend is taking	You do not know what is wrong with her pill, what her friend is taking, what the indications are for another pill, and whether there are any contraindications. There are systems for making the change from one pill to another
I forgot to ask the doctor for some more pills when I came in about my tonsillitis	Many antibiotics reduce the effectiveness of the COC. You do not know how the doctor advised her. She may need emergency contraception
Can I have a pregnancy test?	Many young women ask for a pregnancy test when what they really need is emergency contraception and they do not know how to ask for it
My pill is making me bleed, can you change it?	Sexually transmitted infections are a common cause of bleeding in women taking the pill. Discussion of sexual health issues is an integral part of the contraception consultation. Alternatively, the woman may not be taking her pill correctly

- how appointments are made for fitting implants, IUDs and the IUS
- the fitting of implants, IUDs and the IUS.

PATIENT QUERIES

Apparently simple queries and requests often turn out not to be so simple after all. Practice nurses should always refer the patient on if the question relates to something outside their knowledge and experience. Some examples of the hidden complexities of 'simple' questions are listed in Table 9.1. All require referral to another practitioner.

> **ESSENTIAL SKILLS**
>
> - Knowledge of the most commonly used methods of contraception and how they work
> - Ability to give suitable advice and information to patients
> - Awareness of legal issues, such as consent, under-16 year olds, child protection and confidentiality
> - How to assess and refer patients to the appropriate professional or service

FURTHER READING

Andrews G (ed.). Women's Sexual Health, 2nd edn. London: Baillière Tindall, 2001.

Belfield T. Contraceptive Handbook, 3rd edn. London: Family Planning Association, 1999.

Everett S. Handbook of Contraception and Family Planning. London: Baillière Tindall, 1997.

Guillebaud J. Contraception: Your Questions Answered, 3rd edn. London: Churchill Livingstone, 1999.

Sutherland C. Women's Health: A Handbook for Nurses. Edinburgh: Churchill Livingstone, 2001.

Szarewski A, Guillebaud J. Contraception: A User's Handbook, 3rd edn. Oxford: Oxford University Press, 2002.

White S. Supporting Effective Contraceptive Use: A Resource for Practice Nurses. London: Health Education Authority; 1998.

USEFUL WEBSITES

fpa (formerly the Family Planning Association): leaflets, information packs and other resources. Tel. 01865 719418; http://www.fpa.org.uk

Health Promotion England: closed on the 31 March 2002 and its core functions transferred to the Department of Health on 1 April 2002.

Chapter 10

The menopause

Gilly Andrews

Improved healthcare is increasing life expectancy. As health professionals, we should aim to help women to maximize their postmenopausal health and to lead an active and independent life for as long as possible. As you gain experience in this area of women's health you will be able to offer sound advice, not just about the menopause and associated health issues, but also about lifestyle, non-hormonal therapies and hormone replacement therapy (HRT).

PHYSIOLOGY OF THE MENOPAUSE

The term 'menopause' refers specifically to the end of menstruation, the average age of which is 51 years in the UK. Women who smoke have an earlier menopause, usually before the age of 40 years.

Ovarian function declines during the perimenopausal years and the ovaries eventually fail when they run out of primordial follicles. The terms 'climacteric' or 'perimenopause' refer to the time on either side of the last period. During this transitional phase the ovaries produce less oestrogen, which in turn reduces the negative feedback to the pituitary gland, so follicle-stimulating hormone (FSH) levels begin to rise.

DIAGNOSIS OF THE MENOPAUSE

Women in their forties with vague symptoms or menstrual irregularities will frequently ask, 'Is it the change? Can I have a blood test?' It is rarely useful to perform blood tests as hormone levels can fluctuate widely and are therefore confusing and unreliable. Blood tests (of FSH) are usually only indicated when a premature menopause is suspected, or to exclude conditions that may cause similar symptoms (e.g. anaemia or thyroid disease).

The best way to diagnose the menopause is by taking a thorough history of symptoms and menstrual irregularities. Menopause can only be diagnosed with absolute certainty in retrospect, as ovulation and a period could still occur after many months of amenorrhea.[1] Consequently, it is recommended that women use contraception for 2 years if their last period occurs under the age of 50 years, or for 1 year when it occurs after the age of 50 years.

SYMPTOMS OF THE MENOPAUSE

The fall in oestrogen levels that occurs at the menopause can cause a variety of symptoms (Figure 10.1). Although the list seems alarming, few women experience them all and some women are fortunate enough to have no problems. From a medical perspective, the immediate symptoms are mostly harmless, but it is the longer term consequences of oestrogen deficiency on the skeletal system that cause anxiety.

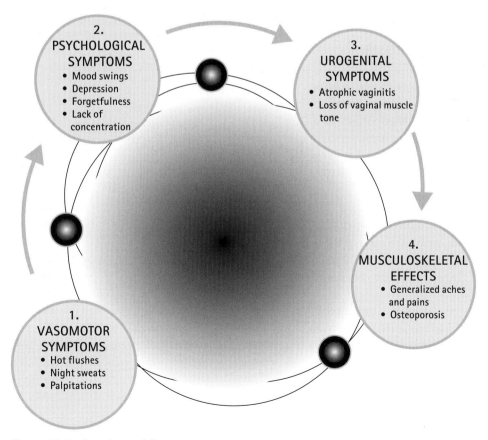

Figure 10.1   Symptoms of the menopause.

The menstrual cycle during the perimenopause is erratic. Some women experience heavy and more frequent bleeding, while others have lighter bleeding with ever-increasing gaps between periods as ovarian function declines.

MENOPAUSE AND HEART DISEASE

Cardiovascular disease (CVD) is unusual before the menopause, but becomes the most common cause of death in women over 50 years old.[2] Until recently it was thought that HRT reduced the incidence of CVD. Recent studies, however, have caused confusion by not showing these benefits for either secondary prevention (i.e. women who already have CVD) or for primary prevention (i.e. women without CVD).[3, 4] HRT is currently not recommended for the prevention of heart disease.

MENOPAUSE AND OSTEOPOROSIS

Bone density gradually declines with age in both men and women, but this loss is more rapid in women after the menopause. Osteoporosis is a condition in which bone mass is reduced to such an extent that fractures may occur following even minimal trauma. There are many risk factors (Box 10.1).

The most common fracture sites are the forearm, spine (leading to the classic 'dowager's hump') and femoral neck. In the UK, one in three women and one in twelve men over the age of 50 years will suffer a fragility fracture caused by osteoporosis.[5]

Osteoporosis not only causes considerable pain, disability and stress to the sufferer, but also has huge financial implications for the NHS.

Testing for osteoporosis

The gold standard for measuring bone density is with a dual energy X-ray absorptiometry (DEXA) scan of the hip and spine. It is not readily available in all areas, but is recommended for those who are at high risk and where results would influence management.

A cheaper way of predicting future osteoporotic fracture risk is by using quantitative ultrasound (QUS) of the heel. Although QUS does not measure bone density directly, it is a useful aid to diagnosis in some situations.

MANAGEMENT STRATEGIES

Some women view the menopause as a positive and fulfilling stage of their lives, with diminishing anxieties about contraception and periods.

BOX 10.1   Risk factors for osteoporosis[6]
Genetic
• Family history (especially mother or sister)
Constitutional
• Low body mass index (BMI)
• Early menopause (under 45 years old)
Environmental
• Cigarette smoking
• Alcohol abuse
• Low calcium intake
• Sedentary lifestyle
Drugs
• Corticosteroids (> 5 mg prednisolone or equivalent daily)
Diseases
• Anorexia nervosa
• Rheumatoid arthritis
• Neuromuscular disease
• Chronic liver disease
• Malabsorption syndromes
• Hyperthyroidism
• Hyperparathyroidism

Others, however, are less positive and may ask your advice. It is a good idea if this information can be given proactively while a woman is in her 40s (at smear tests and contraceptive checks), and not just when she starts experiencing symptoms.

When discussing the menopause it is important to spend time explaining the nature of the symptoms, the possible long-term consequences on health and the treatment options available. If possible, it helps women make informed decisions if you can back up information with leaflets.

HORMONE REPLACEMENT THERAPY

HRT relieves menopausal symptoms and improves bone density.

If a woman has had a hysterectomy she need only take oestrogen for HRT. However, if she has a uterus then she must take progestogen as well as oestrogen, as this prevents the endometrium from becoming too thick (endometrial hyperplasia).

Progestogen can be added to oestrogen in three ways (Figure 10.2):

- sequentially – which will give a monthly period

- tricyclically – which should give a period every 3 months
- continuously – giving a 'period-free' option. This is suitable only for women who are at least 1 year postmenopausal, otherwise irregular bleeding can occur.

A gonadomimetic is similar to a continuous combined preparation. The intrauterine system (Mirena) can also be used for the progestogen component of HRT. It is not yet licensed for this use in the UK, but has such a licence in other countries. It has the additional advantages of providing contraception for the perimenopausal woman and making periods substantially lighter.

There are a number of different routes of administration for HRT:

- oral
- transdermal
- patches
- gel
- intranasal
- implant
- vaginal (available for urogenital symptom relief only, or for systemic symptoms).

For most women it makes little difference which route is chosen, and patient preference may be the determining factor. If a woman has a pre-existing

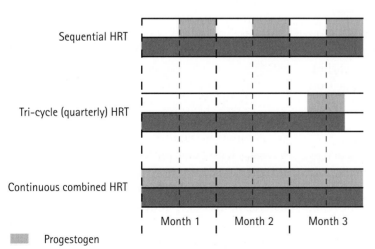

Figure 10.2   Oestrogen/progestogen preparations for women with a uterus.

medical condition it might be better to avoid the '-first-pass' effect of the liver with oral preparations and use a transdermal preparation instead.[6]

Despite the benefits of HRT (Box 10.2) uptake remains low. Many women have been alarmed about potential risks (Box 10.3) and they might seek your advice about whether to start HRT, or change or discontinue their current preparation. In order to make sure that the information you give is unbiased and accurate it is important to keep yourself regularly updated with current research and management strategies so that you can help women make informed decisions.

NON-HORMONAL ALTERNATIVES

For osteoporosis

- Bisphosphonates prevent and treat osteoporosis.
- Selective oestrogen receptor modulators (SERMs) act as oestrogen does on the bone without stimulating breast or endometrial tissue.
- Calcium and vitamin D: it is not clear whether the bone benefits are because of vitamin D, calcium, or a combination of both.

For general well-being

Some women do not wish to take any medication to help them through what they perceive as a natural transitional phase and try other approaches. The following therapies are popular, but you should mention to women who seek your advice that they are expensive and there is scant evidence for their efficacy.

Phyto-oestrogens found in soy products (such as red clover) are meant to have a weak estrogenic effect.

Natural progesterone creams may give some relief for hot flushes, but should not be used for the progestogen element of HRT, as they do not give enough endometrial protection.

> **BOX 10.2   Benefits of HRT**
>
> - Improvement of menopausal symptoms
> - Decrease in osteoporotic fractures
> - Reduction in colorectal cancer
> - Less depression
> - Improved sexuality and libido
> - Improved quality/length of life

> **BOX 10.3   Risks of HRT**
>
> - Increase in breast cancer with over 5 years of use. The number of cases per 1,000 women would rise from 45 to 47 (i.e. by 2). This risk returns to normal within 5 years of stopping HRT[7]
> - Increase in venous thromboembolism in first year of use from one per 10,000 to three per 10,000[8]
> - Increase in CVD[4] (although some clinicians feel these studies were flawed as many of the recruited women were not healthy menopausal women but older with coexisting medical problems)
> - Increase in endometrial cancer if progestogen is not added for women with a uterus

---

Nutritional therapies in the form of additional vitamins and minerals are thought unnecessary if a well balanced diet is eaten.

Herbal remedies are not subject to the same regulations as drugs and it is difficult to know what some preparations may contain; they can interfere with other prescribed medication. There is little research to show there is any benefit.

Other complementary therapies, such as aromatherapy, massage, reflexology, yoga and acupuncture, have been found useful in relieving some menopausal symptoms, particularly those associated with stress.

HEALTHY LIFESTYLE ADVICE

Healthy lifestyle advice is important at all stages in life, but is particularly relevant for the older woman when the incidence of CVD increases. All the following strategies improve general health and are evidence-based at reducing CVD:

> ### ESSENTIAL SKILLS
>
> - Understand the physiology of the menopause, and its diagnosis and symptoms
> - Understand the issues surrounding heart disease and osteoporosis with respect to the menopause
> - Keep up to date with research and management strategies
> - Provide advice and information opportunistically to women in their 40s and older
> - Understand the risks and benefits of HRT and other treatment options
> - Encourage a healthy lifestyle

- stop smoking
- drink alcohol in moderation
- eat a healthy, well-balanced diet with the recommended 700 mg calcium intake
- exercise regularly (weight-bearing exercise is good for the skeletal system as it maintains bone strength and improves agility, therefore reducing falls and fractures).

Women should be encouraged to be breast aware and have regular mammograms and cervical smears.

CONCLUSION

Nurses have an important role to play in the management of the menopause. Women often prefer talking to their practice nurse rather than the doctor. You can be the linchpin in running an efficient and effective menopause service for the benefit of both colleagues and patients.

REFERENCES

1. Burger HG. The endocrinology of the menopause. J Steroid Biochem 1999; 69: 31–35.
2. Mortality Statistics Sause Review of the Registrar General on Deaths by Cause, Sex and Age, in England and Wales 1999: Series DH2 No. 26. London: Office for National Statistics. Available at: http://www.statistics.gov.uk
3. Hully S, Grady D, Bush T, et al. Randomised trial of estrogen and progestin for secondary prevention of coronary heart disease in postmenopausal women. JAMA 1998; 280: 605–612.
4. Writing Group for the Women's Health Initiative Investigators. Risks and benefits of estrogen plus progestin in healthy postmenopausal women: principal results from the Women's Health Initiative randomized controlled trial. JAMA 2002; 288: 321–333.
5. Torgerson DJ, Iglesias CP, Reid DM. The economics of fracture prevention. In: Barlow DH, Francis RM, Miles A (eds). The Effective Management of Osteoporosis. London: Aesculapius Medical Press, 2001.
6. Rees M, Purdie DW (eds). Management of the Menopause. The Handbook of the British Menopause Society 2002. Marlow: BMS Publications, 2002.
7. Collaborative Group on Hormonal Factors in Breast Cancer. Breast cancer and HRT: collaborative reanalysis of data from 51 epidemiological studies. Lancet 1997; 330: 1047–1059.
8. Lowe G, Woodward M, Vessey M, et al. Thrombotic variables and risk of idiopathic venous thromboembolism in women aged 45–64 years. Relationships to HRT. Thrombosis Haemostas 2000; 83: 530–535.

Chapter 11

Men's health

Jane DeVille-Almond

Men still die earlier than women on average, and have higher rates of just about every common disease. Yet most general practices ignore gender differences when planning their services.

The issue was highlighted in 1993, when the Chief Medical Officer's annual general report urged health authorities to investigate ways of promoting men's health.[1] As well as male-specific illnesses such as prostate disorders, the document identified coronary heart disease, cancers, sexual health, accidents, suicide, and mental health problems as being particular concerns for men.

Many primary care staff, from the receptionist to the doctor, see patients as genderless. They tend to have a 'take it or leave it' attitude – so if men don't want to use primary care services that is their choice.

Take a look around your waiting room. How inviting and friendly is it for young and middle-aged men? My bet is that there are few posters on male issues, no male reading material, and that the opening times are most suited to housewives and the elderly. Now think about how you might change this, and how you could remember gender differences when dealing with patients.

MAKE A DIFFERENCE

Audit your male patients

It really is worth taking a look at the demographics of your practice. Check how many male and how many female patients you have, then break down the male group by age. This will give you an idea of the type of services you should consider offering.

If you have a high proportion of men over 50 years of age you might consider putting on a talk one evening about prostate awareness. If you have a high proportion of young men you might want to arrange an open day with information and an open-access clinic. Discuss these ideas with your practice team.

Surgery times

How many men find it difficult to make an appointment at the surgery because of the opening times? You may think that if a man is ill enough he will have to make the effort to fit in with the times on offer. However, this can lead to delays, and a relatively minor illness may become more serious.[2-6] Think about offering men a questionnaire asking if the opening times are convenient, and whether they would prefer to attend surgeries in the evening, early morning or Saturday.

Posters and leaflets

Look at your poster displays. It might be a good idea to focus on men's health occasionally, perhaps dedicating a whole area to the subject.

Perhaps you could set up a special corner devoted to men's health, where male-specific literature can be displayed. This might make it easier for men to collect information on potentially embarrassing conditions rather than having to take leaflets from a stand in full view of everyone – as is often the case.

Consider making up information packs aimed at specific age groups. A folder for young men could offer literature on issues such as sexual health, testicular awareness, and depression. Older men could be given a package on prostate disorders, sexual dysfunction, and bladder problems. Clearly there are more common health

problems, but these are topics that men tend to feel most embarrassed about, and may not want to pick up the relevant leaflets from a shelf in the waiting room.

Protocols for medicals

Do you have a protocol specifically for men? Many of the protocols in current use are not specific to either sex. However, it is important to use routine health checks as an opportunity to discuss, offer information about, and record problems specific to men's health. These issues include:

- history of testicular problems
- history of prostate problems
- erectile dysfunction
- bowel habits
- depression.

When you conduct a new patient medical for a man who has registered with the practice, remember you probably will not see him again until he is ill. It is essential to use this initial consultation to instil confidence and encourage good communication for the future, as well as to collect standard health information.

KEY CONDITIONS

Some of the conditions that have important implications for men's health are considered embarrassing and difficult to discuss. You need to be able to ask the right questions and offer appropriate advice.

Bowel disorders

The patient needs to understand why you are asking about his bowel habits, and what the significance might be.

The most common bowel problems include constipation and diarrhoea, Crohn's disease and ulcerative colitis, haemorrhoids (piles), and bowel cancer.

Bowel cancer is the third most common malignancy in the UK, with more than 30,000 new cases annually. It is a little more common in men than women, and kills about 17,000 people each year. The symptoms are similar to those of many non-life-threatening conditions, but it is important for the patient to know what they are so he can obtain early intervention. Changes that might suggest bowel cancer include:

- any change in bowel habits, such as bouts of constipation or diarrhoea
- bleeding from the rectum, either dark blood mixed with stools or bright red blood
- abdominal pain
- weight loss
- poor appetite
- a lump in the abdomen
- tiredness (this may be a sign of anaemia).

Depression

Depression is very common and can affect anyone – male or female, young or old. However, the rate of depression appears to be increasing among men and decreasing among women. More worryingly, suicide is now the most common cause of death in England in men under 35 years old, and the rate of suicide in men aged 15–24 years has more than doubled since 1971.[4]

Depression is a complex disorder, with many different risk factors. We can all feel a little down from time to time, but if this persists it could be a sign of depression. Your patient may need help if he has five or more of the following symptoms:[5]

- persistent feeling of sadness or unhappiness, often worse at particular times of the day, especially early morning
- loss of interest in pleasure or life
- inappropriate feelings of guilt
- feeling worthless
- difficulties with concentration and memory
- loss of appetite

- significant unplanned weight loss
- sleeping difficulties such as early waking or problems falling asleep
- thoughts of suicide.

Erectile dysfunction

Most men experience an erection problem at least once in their lives, often caused by stress, too much alcohol, or simply just not feeling like sex. Persistent erectile dysfunction is estimated to affect around one in ten men, and the risk increases with advancing age.

Erectile dysfunction is not life-threatening, but it can be very distressing, and often leads to depression and relationship problems if not treated. It may also be an early sign of more serious conditions, such as diabetes or heart disease. It is important to give the man an opportunity to discuss erectile dysfunction and to seek advice. There are several treatments available for erectile dysfunction, which the man should discuss with his doctor.

Prostate conditions

About 50% of men will develop prostate disease at some time in their lives, with most of these suffering with benign prostatic hyperplasia. The risk of this increases with age.

Prostate cancer is the second most common cause of cancer-related death in British men.[6] During 2003 it affected about 24,000 men in the UK and killed about 10,000. Many men do not even know where or what the prostate is, so information should be available on the subject.

There are also prostate conditions that affect younger men, including prostatitis. Men of all ages need to understand that they should consult their GP if they experience any of the classic prostate symptoms:

- having to get up during the night to urinate, often more than once

- feeling that the bladder is not completely empty after going to the toilet
- sometimes having to go to the toilet again in less than 2 hours
- stopping and starting several times when going to the toilet
- having a weak stream of urine
- slight urinary incontinence and an inability to hold on to urine
- difficulty with urination, needing to strain or push.

Testicular awareness

Although testicular cancer is not common, its incidence has doubled over the past two decades. There were about 1,500 cases in 2003 in the UK.[7] It is a disease that predominantly affects young men between the ages of 15 and 40 years, and it is life-threatening if not detected and treated promptly. However, therapeutic advances, particularly in chemotherapy, mean that effective treatment is available for cases that are diagnosed in time. Survival is now over 90%.

It is important to advise men to report any changes immediately, including new lumps, bumps, aches, pains, or changes in size. Although advice on testicular awareness should be given to men of all ages, it may be worth explaining to men over 50 years old that the condition is extremely rare in this age group.

ENCOURAGE DISCUSSION

Discussing such a wide range of subjects may seem difficult at first, but once you are familiar with these areas and learn how to handle potentially embarrassing issues these consultations will become second nature.

Sometimes it is more effective to offer information rather than ask a direct question. For example, you might say 'Erectile dysfunction affects 1 in 10 men at some point in their lives, and did you know it could be the first sign of some other condition such as heart disease or diabetes?' This shows the patient that you are not worried about discussing erectile dysfunction, and it enables him to continue the conversation. This technique can be used with other topics such as depression, where you can mention that some depressions cannot be treated without medical intervention, so it is important to seek help early.

Because many men do not use general practice in the same way as women they often do not understand what the roles of the nurse and GP are. It is important to reassure the patient that by coming in with a condition in its early stages he might be preventing it getting worse, and is not wasting anyone's time.

CONCLUSION

Gender differences do exist, and it is important to offer services that meet the needs of male patients. It also means that everyone in the practice team, including the receptionists, has to understand that they may need to take a different approach with patients, depending on their sex.

There are many new books available on men's health, and it is well worth getting some for your surgery, for you and your colleagues, and for patients to borrow if necessary.

ESSENTIAL SKILLS

- Understanding and minimizing the barriers to promoting men's health
- Incorporating male-specific issues into new patient consultations
- Advising patients on the main health issues, such as bowel disorders, depression, erectile dysfunction, prostate conditions, and coronary heart disease
- Promoting testicular awareness
- Adopting a consultation technique to help men discuss potentially embarrassing topics

REFERENCES

1. Calman K. Chief Medical Officer's Annual Report 1993. London: Department of Health, 1993.
2. Davidson N, Lloyd T. Promoting Men's Health – A Guide for Practitioners. London: Baillière Tindall, 2001.
3. Men's Health Forum, Tackling men's health inequalities. 2001. Available at: http://www.menshealthforum.org.uk
4. Men's Health Forum, Solder it! Young men and suicide. Available at: http://www.menshealthforum.org.uk
5. http://www.malehealth.co.uk
6. Kirby RS, Kirby MG, Farah RN. Men's Health. Oxford: Isis Medical Media, 1999.
7. Mens Health Forum, Getting it sorted: a new policy for men's heath, a consultative document. Available at: http://www.menshealthforum.org.uk

FURTHER READING

Banks I. Ask Dr Ian About Men's Health. Belfast: Blackstaff Press, 1997.

Banks I. The Haynes Man Manual. Somerset: Haynes, 2002.

O'Dowd T, Jewell D, Men's Health. Oxford: Oxford University Press, 1998.

USEFUL WEBSITES

Fatmanslim gives weight management advice specifically focused on men: http://www.fatmanslim.co.uk

Men's Health Forum: http://www.menshealthforum.org.uk

LEAFLETS AND POSTERS

Life begins at 40 – health tips for men (Department of Health/Health Promotion Resources, http://www.dh.gov.uk)

Are you too shy to talk about number 2 (Tel. 020 8892 5256, e-mail: info@beatingbowelcancer.org)

Beating bowel cancer (Tel. 020 8892 5256, e-mail: info@beatingbowelcancer.org)

Testicular cancer. Spot the symptoms early (Cancer Research UK, Tel. 08701 555 455, e-mail: doh@prolog.uk.com (quote 27036 testicular cancer))

Waterworks problems? Don't suffer in silence (Tel. 020 8332 7608, website: http://www.mhm.tv)

Men's health matters (Tel. 020 8332 7608, website: http://www.mhm.tv)

The prostate gland owner's manual (The Prostate Cancer Charity, Tel. 020 8222 7622, e-mail: literature@prostate-cancer.org.uk)

Prostate cancer: the works (The Prostate Cancer Charity, Tel. 020 8222 7622, e-mail: literature@prostate-cancer.org.uk)

The prostate cancer tool kit (The Prostate Cancer Charity, Tel. 020 8222 7622, e-mail: literature@prostate-cancer.org.uk)

Manmatters: information and advice on erection problems (Tel. 0800 096 4348, website: http://www.manmatters.netdoctor.co.uk)

Chapter 12

Men and sexual health

Jane DeVille-Almond

England is witnessing a rapid decline in sexual health (Box 12.1). The prevalence of sexually transmitted infections (STIs) is increasing dramatically, and the number of visits to genito-urinary medicine (GUM) clinics has doubled over the past decade to exceed a million a year.[1,2] These infections can have long-term effects on people's lives.

The first national strategy for sexual health and the human immunodeficiency virus (HIV) was

---

BOX 12.1   STI facts and figures

- There was an 84% increase in gonorrhoea in England between 1997 and 2001
- Syphilis has increased more than six-fold, but remains relatively rare
- More than 29,000 male patients were diagnosed with *Chlamydia* in 2001, making this the most common curable bacterial STI
- By the end of 2002 more than 54,000 people in the UK had been diagnosed with HIV, 77% of them male
- Waiting times for GUM appointments for males increased from 5 days in 2001 to 12 days in 2002
- Sexual health services such as community family planning clinics are underused by men. More than 12 times as many women as men attended in 1999–2000

launched in July 2001, with the aims of modernizing services, addressing the rising prevalence and exploring the impact on public health.[2] It states:

> Sexual health is an important part of physical and mental health. It is a key part of our identity as human beings together with the fundamental human right to privacy, a family life and living free from discrimination. Essential elements of good sexual health are equitable relationships and sexual fulfilment with access to information and services to avoid the risk of unintended pregnancy, illness or disease.

The strategy describes the significant variations in the quality of sexual health services across the country as unacceptable. It calls for standards to be improved in line with the principles set out in the NHS Plan.

BARRIERS TO CARE

Sexuality and sexual health are appropriate and legitimate aspects of nursing care. Nurses have a professional obligation to address them. Some nurses, particularly those new to general practice, can find the subject embarrassing, for reasons such as:[3]

- inadequate education about sexual health and sexuality at both pre-registration and post-registration levels
- personal views, for example a belief that homosexuality is wrong or religious taboos against contraception
- a belief that sexuality and sexual health are not important or not appropriate in certain circumstances, such as in care of the elderly
- lack of confidence.

GETTING STARTED

It is important for new practice nurses to familiarize themselves with the practice policy on STIs. Where there is no policy, they should make sure one is drafted.

It may be difficult to raise the subject of STIs with a male patient. Just talking generally around the subject and offering information for future reading may be an ideal way of introducing the topic.

The practice needs to have information specifically aimed at men. This can be obtained through primary care trust health promotion units and various STI-related organizations. This literature could be included in the pack given out to men at new-patient medicals or other routine consultations.

Practice nurses need to be particularly sensitive when dealing with STIs. Patients are often extremely embarrassed or feel guilty, especially where one partner may infect the other. There is still a social stigma attached to STIs, so patients often need to be reassured about confidentiality.

GUM CLINICS

We have come a long way since the treatments for STIs included cold baths, wrapping the sex organs in wool and abstinence from sexual intercourse. However, many GUM clinics are still tucked away in basements or at the rear of the hospital, reinforcing the idea that sexual health should not be talked about in public.[3]

GUM staff are specially trained to deal with STIs and have all the relevant diagnostic equipment on site. Patients attending a GUM clinic do not need to give their full name or real name if they do not wish to, and no other details will be taken against the patient's wishes.

Practice nurses should make sure they have the telephone number and address of their local GUM clinic to hand. They can then make appointments or give out the number so patients can make arrangements for themselves. A few GUM clinics offer a walk-in service, so make sure you know what is available in your area.

Even if an appointment is made in the surgery, it is difficult to know for certain whether the patient will attend. The practice nurse must reiterate the importance of seeking treatment and informing partners.

CHLAMYDIA

Chlamydial infection is the most common curable STI in the developed world. The incidence rose by 20% between 1999 and 2000. Although this may be attributed to better screening services, it is more likely to indicate a rise in the number of people practising unsafe sex.[3]

Many cases of *Chlamydia* remain undetected, with half of those men infected remaining asymptomatic. Many men have never even heard of the condition. The good news is that condoms provide almost total protection.

Chlamydia causes few problems for men, but the consequences can be disastrous if the infection is passed on to women. The organism is not only the single biggest cause of infection of the fallopian tubes, leading to infertility and ectopic pregnancy, it can also cause blindness and pneumonia in a child born to an infected woman.

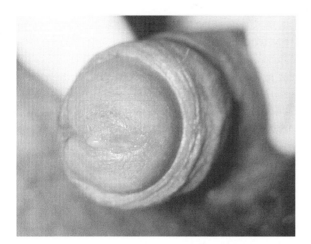

Figure 12.1 Urethritis, with penile discharge and dysuria, caused by chlamydial infection.

Signs and symptoms

Men infected with *Chlamydia* may complain of:

- a burning sensation when passing urine
- a white discharge (Figure 12.1)
- general symptoms, such as abdominal pain, rash and joint pains.

There are many tests available for *Chlamydia*, but as yet no single investigation will identify all cases. All the tests require a urine sample.

Treatment

Chlamydia is treated with the antibiotic azithromycin, which can be prescribed by the GP or at the GUM clinic.

PENILE WARTS

One in eight people attending the GUM clinic have genital warts.[4] These are caused by the papilloma viruses, which can affect any part of the skin. Penile warts are exactly like the warts commonly seen on hands, and their size can range from a tiny skin tag to a large mass.

Some strains of the papilloma virus are associated with cervical cancer, and can therefore be dangerous if passed on to female partners.

Signs and symptoms

Warts are seen or felt on the penis. They may be itchy, leading to scratching and bleeding. Otherwise they generally cause little discomfort.

Treatment

Various creams can be prescribed. These are applied directly to the wart, causing it to disappear. In some cases the creams act by burning the wart off. Choice of treatment depends on the size and site of the wart. Although it is possible to get over-the-counter treatments, it is always advisable to consult a GP or nurse first.

Condoms prevent transmission of warts, and are a useful way of avoiding the virus.

HERPES SIMPLEX

Genital herpes is the third most common STI, and is currently incurable. It is caused by the herpes simplex virus (HSV), which comes in two forms, HSV 1 and HSV 2. Both infect parts of the body where two types of skin meet, such as the corner of the mouth and the outer genital areas.[4]

Bouts of herpes simplex can last for months, then disappear for years. Sometimes the condition never returns. When the sores are present they are definitely infectious, but it is still possible to catch the virus when no sores are apparent. The sores often return at times of stress or during illnesses that lower the body's resistance.

Signs and symptoms

Patients experience tingling, itch and a painful sensation in the affected area. Crusted blisters form, that often burn and itch, similar to cold sores on the lips. In later stages, the blisters weep a thin, watery substance, which is highly infectious, as it contains the herpes virus.

Treatment

Antiviral drugs such as aciclovir can be taken orally or applied directly to the skin. They are most effective before the sores break out, so patients should be advised to seek medical attention as soon as they feel the tingling sensation.

During an attack, patients should avoid intercourse and oral sex. During periods of respite, sufferers should always use condoms. Those with spermicide appear to offer greater protection.[3]

GONORRHOEA

Gonorrhoea is caused by a bacterium. It is common and extremely contagious. The incubation period is relatively short – some symptoms can occur within 24 hours of infection.

Signs and symptoms

Men with gonorrhoea experience pain on passing urine and may have a yellow/white discharge from the penis. Other symptoms include vague aching of the joints and muscles and urethritis.

Oral sex with an infected partner may lead to pyrexia, lymphadenopathy and tonsillitis. Anal sex with an infected partner may lead to mild anal pruritus, mucopurulent rectal discharge or slight bleeding, severe rectal pain, constipation and tenesmus (a painful ineffectual straining to empty the bowel).

Most of the symptoms start within 3–5 days of infection and may disappear after a further 10 days or so. Even without symptoms, the patient remains infected until treated.

Treatment

An antibiotic, usually azithromycin, is the usual treatment. If gonorrhoea is left untreated, the patient may suffer from reduced fertility. Condoms provide almost 100% protection against infection.[3]

SYPHILIS

Although the incidence of syphilis has risen more than six-fold, the condition remains relatively rare. It is caused by a highly infectious microscopic parasite. Most people are unaware of the infection and it can develop over several years into a condition that affects the brain.

Signs and symptoms

A small, painless red macule appears during the early stages of the disease. If it is left untreated the macule heals spontaneously in about 3 weeks, but further symptoms may develop 1–3 months after the initial infection. At this stage the patient may complain of:

- flu-like symptoms
- anorexia
- sore throat
- malaise
- lymphadenopathy
- hair loss
- rash on several sites, including palms, soles and trunk.

Treatment

An injection of penicillin is given if the condition is diagnosed in the early stages of development, and a regimen of penicillin injections is used thereafter, depending on the disease and the clinician in charge of treatments. Condoms give almost 100% protection.

HEPATITIS B

Hepatitis B is one of the most deadly STIs, but it can be prevented by vaccination. Patients should be offered the vaccine if their lifestyle puts them at risk (e.g. known drug addicts, patients who have had unprotected sex with multiple partners).

The hepatitis B virus is transmitted intravenously or subcutaneously, which means people are at greater risk if they receive blood or share needles. The virus is also present in body fluids

such as saliva, urine and semen, so it tends to spread through close personal contact such as sexual intercourse, especially anal, and in areas of overcrowding, poverty, and poor sanitation. Piercing and tattooing can also spread the virus. The incubation period is about 2–6 months.[5]

HIV INFECTION

The incidence of HIV infection continues to rise, with more than 4,000 new cases reported each year and perhaps 10 times this number going unrecognized.

In the UK, 77% of the 54,000 known HIV patients are male, something that practice nurses should bear in mind when giving sexual health advice in the surgery.

The first stage of HIV infection is often through exchange of body fluids with an infected individual. Unprotected vaginal or anal intercourse is the most common route of transmission. There have been reports of infection via other intimate sexual activities such as oral sex, but it is difficult to determine whether the virus is transmitted this way, as such acts do not often occur in isolation.[6]

Other routes of transmission are through blood, both transfusions and sharing of equipment, piercing procedures and tattoos, and from mother to child.[5]

GAY MEN

Men who have sex with other men are at an increased risk of STIs. This includes men who identify themselves as gay, but also men who do not, but who still engage in sex with other men.[7]

It can often be difficult for a nurse to discuss the sexual behaviour of men, and for patients to bring up the subject. It is important not to make assumptions or ask closed questions such as 'What does your girlfriend think?' or 'Have you discussed it with your wife?', as this may deter the man from telling his full history in case it embarrasses the nurse.

It is important to remember that not all gay men face the same risks. Many are in long-term, monogamous relationships.[7]

As well as having higher rates of the conditions conventionally classified as STIs, such as syphilis, gonorrhoea and *Chlamydia*, gay men may also contract other sexually encountered infections, such as enteric bacteria, parasites and viruses.

There may be non-infectious problems, such as trauma to the anus or rectum and allergies to lubricants. Trauma can produce mucosal tears and fissures, leading to inflammation, bleeding, rectal pain, burning and mucopurulent discharge, similar to those encountered with STIs.

FURTHER INFORMATION

If you are new to practice nursing there are a number of useful resources and websites available that advise on men's sexual health (see below). In particular, a report from the Men's Health Forum, published in June 2003, highlighted poor services for sexual health.[1] This report aims to increase awareness and knowledge, and encourage men to seek advice or treatment when appropriate. It also offers encouragement to nurses and other service providers to promote and develop more effective, male-friendly sexual health policies and services.[1]

ESSENTIAL SKILLS

- Make yourself aware of your practice policy for STIs
- Know the telephone number and address of your local GUM clinic
- Know how the GUM clinic appointment system works – walk in or appointment only?
- Have appropriate literature available
- Be open and aware during a consultation – do not make assumptions

---

REFERENCES

1. Men's Health Forum. Private Parts, Public Policy – Improving Men's Sexual Health. London: MHF, 2003.
2. Department of Health. National Strategy for Sexual Health and HIV. London: TSO, 2001.
3. Peate I. Men's Sexual Health. London: Whurr, 2003.
4. Banks I. Man: Haynes Owners Workshop Manual. Yeovil: Haynes, 2002.
5. Alexander MF, Fawcett JN, Runciman PJ. Nursing Practice: Hospital and Home – the Adult, 2nd edn. London: Churchill Livingstone, 2000.
6. Rothenberg RB, Scarlett M, del Rio C, Rezmik D, O'Daniels C. Oral transmission of AIDS. AIDS 1998; 12: 2095–2105.
7. Kirby RS, Kirby MG, Farah RN. Men's Health. Oxford: Isis Medical Media, 1999.

USEFUL WEBSITES

Men's Health Forum: http://www.menshealthforum.org.uk

Malehealth: http://www.malehealth.co.uk

Department of Health: http://www.dh.gov.uk

Chapter 13

Health promotion

Tina Bishop

The World Health Organization (WHO) defines health as:

> The extent to which an individual or group is able, on the one hand, to realize aspirations and satisfy needs; and on the other hand, to change or cope with the environment. Health is therefore seen as a resource for everyday life, not an object of living; it is a positive concept emphasizing social and personal resources, as well as physical capacities.

'Health promotion' is a widely used term among healthcare professionals, encompassing many concepts and ideas. It originated in the 19th century when infectious diseases, which spread in the overcrowded industrial towns, were the big killers. Pressure for reform led to public health legislation to educate people in how to avoid contracting these diseases. However, it was improved living conditions, sanitation and diet that brought about a real reduction in their spread.

Health promotion is often viewed as synonymous with health education – after all if you educate people (i.e. tell them what to do) they can avoid illness and disease and be healthy. However, as Professor Keith Tones points out, health promotion is a broader concept that 'incorporates all measures deliberately designed to promote health and handle disease'. A 'healthy public policy' can achieve social change with legislation.[1]

DEFINITIONS OF HEALTH

'Health' is another broad term that means different things to individuals at different stages of their lives. An average person may define health as being physically fit and not being ill. Academics such as Professor David Seedhouse suggest that health is a foundation for human achievement, enabling people to reach their full potential.[2] The WHO definition (see p. 75) encompasses this idea, establishing health as a social product, and emphasizing the dynamic and positive nature of health.[3, 4]

Influences on health

There are many factors that influence health and well-being, including social class, gender, housing, employment and poverty. How much money you have greatly influences your life expectations and choices, and also your health status.

HEALTH PROMOTION IN PRACTICE

Primary healthcare is the first level of contact that the public usually have with the NHS. An estimated 97% of the population is registered with a GP and over 75% will consult a GP at least once a year.[4] As well as GPs, general practice also enables patients to gain access to practice nurses, health visitors, chiropodists and counsellors, and would therefore seem an ideal place to promote health through planned strategies or opportunistic interventions.

Types of health promotion advice

Health promotion in general practice usually takes a medical focus, which aims to limit/prevent illness and premature death, and is usually considered within the following framework.

- *Primary health promotion* is prevention of diseases and illness, for example through immunization, promoting a healthy lifestyle and screening for early detection and prevention of disease (e.g. cervical cytology, and advising patients about breast awareness and testicular self-examination).
- *Secondary health promotion* aims to shorten or prevent episodes of illness and chronic disease such as asthma or diabetes.
- *Tertiary health promotion* is aimed at prevention, to reduce further disability and complications arising from irreversible conditions such as heart disease and stroke.

Models for health promotion

Both opportunistic (unplanned) and planned models of promoting health take place in general practice. Opportunistic health promotion is usually added onto a consultation, where appropriate (e.g. discussing sexual health issues when taking a cervical smear). Planned health promotion is where patients are attending the practice for predetermined preventive healthcare (e.g. an immunization clinic).

There is some indication that opportunistic health promotion is more effective than planned interventions.[5] However, time constraints are an issue and there are ethical concerns about informed consent.

Many practice nurses manage a caseload that may include chronic-disease management, running immunization clinics, providing screening sessions, and supporting patients to consider their lifestyle and the choices they make. They can also provide information on a one-to-one basis, or by handing out leaflets and introducing patients to other healthcare workers and self-help groups.

Social and environmental dimensions to health have to be acknowledged. For example, unemployment and poverty are outside the control of the individual, but do have an influence on people's behaviour and the choices they make. Advising someone to buy more fruit may make good sense, but for a mother with two or three children and on a limited income this may not be an option.

THE CHALLENGES

Healthy lifestyles are seen as key to good health. Smoking, poor diet, alcohol intake above the recommended maximum and lack of exercise are all implicated in the development of the major killer diseases of today – coronary heart disease and cancer.

In the past we often blamed people for not taking expert advice and therefore contributing to their own poor health. However, it is worth noting that people can be at risk of heart disease even before they are born – low birth weight and low weight gain in the first year of life are strongly associated with heart disease, and are linked to poverty.

THE GOVERNMENT'S AGENDA

Health promotion programmes can sometimes widen inequalities because the better off make more use of preventive services. The Government strategy for England, *Our Healthier Nation*, aims to improve the health of the worse off and narrow the health divide between the socio-economic groups.[6] The main targets of this strategy are to:

- prevent accidents
- improve mental health services and reduce the incidence of suicides
- reduce the incidence of coronary heart disease and stroke
- reduce the incidence of cancers.

A community approach is seen as the best way to achieve better health in the population. Primary healthcare trusts, together with individual practices, have the responsibility to profile their community in order to identify needs, and then to work across the NHS and other organizations to provide services to meet health needs. Health improvement plans (HImPs) are action plans that must be developed by primary care organizations, health authorities, etc., to identify and address priorities (Box 13.1).

National service frameworks (NSFs) form one of a range of measures to raise quality and decrease variations in services in different regions. They set national guidelines that are

---

> **BOX 13.1 Four strategic themes of a health improvement programme[7]**
>
> - Public health and inequalities in health
> - Range and location of health and relevant social services
> - Government medium-term financial strategy for public services
> - Involving patients and the public in planning and monitoring services

---

TABLE 13.1 Examples of barriers to healthy eating and interventions to address them[8]	
Barrier	**Intervention**
Belief that the family is already eating enough fruit and vegetables	Information about five portions a day and portion size
Dislike of taste of vegetables and lack of confidence in cooking and preparation	Set up cooking skills club and tasting sessions as part of existing groups
Difficulty in finding affordable good quality fruit and vegetables	Set up community owned retailing and food cooperatives

monitored on a regular basis. Strategies to promote health are generally set at several levels in order to identify barriers to health promotion (Table 13.1).

AUDIT OF SERVICES

Audit and evaluation of services is an essential part of the cost- and quality-conscious NHS. Many health promotion services in general practice, such as immunization and cervical smear clinics, are linked to additional service payments, and therefore keeping numbers up can take priority.

If people do not attend services, you need to ask three key questions:

- Is the service run at the right time of day?
- Is transport and getting to the practice an issue?
- Is the service publicized?

CONCLUSION

Promoting health is a complex issue and the practice nurse needs to be aware of all factors that impinge on the process. As well as having and imparting knowledge and information about preventing ill health, nurses also need to collaborate with other agencies to develop services that meet the needs of patients in their community. Ongoing education and development is essential to ensure that services continue to meet the needs of the practice population.

ESSENTIAL SKILLS

- Understand what is meant by primary, secondary and tertiary health promotion
- Recognize and use the opportunities for basic opportunistic health promotion, such as diet, alcohol consumption, smoking cessation and exercise advice
- Undertake basic planned health promotion, such as immunization and new-patient screening
- Provide patient advice and information
- Be familiar with HImPs and the relevant national service frameworks
- Recognize the influences on individual patient health and the potential barriers to change
- Link with the primary care organization to profile the practice population and identify need

REFERENCES

1. Tones K. Why theorise? Ideology in health education. Health Educ J 1990; 44: 4.
2. Seedhouse D. Health: A Foundation for Achievement. Chichester: John Wiley, 1986.
3. World Health Organization. Health Promotion; A Discussion Document on the Concept and Principles. Copenhagen: WHO for Europe, 1984.
4. Naido J, Wills J. Health Promotion, Foundations for Practice, 2nd edn. London: Baillière Tindall, 2000.
5. Doyle Y, Thomas P. Promoting health through primary care: challenges in taking a strategic approach. Health Educ J 1996; 55: 3–10.
6. Department of Health. Our Healthier Nation, Reducing Health Inequalities; An Action Report. London: DoH, 1997.
7. Baker M. What's it all about? Nursing Standard 2000; 14(16): 25.
8. NHS Health Development Agency. Coronary Heart Disease, Guidance for Implementing the Preventive Aspects of the National Service Frameworks. London: NHS; 2001.

FURTHER READING

Carey L (ed.). Practice Nursing. London: Baillière Tindall, 2000. Explores the role of the practice nurse and the issues that impact upon the nursing care they provide.

Chapter 14

Smoking cessation

Jennifer Percival

Smoking is the greatest single cause of preventable illness and premature death in the UK, killing over 120,000 people each year.[1] As most smokers are reluctant to associate such high risk with themselves, this issue needs to be addressed at every opportunity in primary care.

The aim of this chapter is to provide new practice nurses with an insight into how and when to offer advice to smokers, by identifying a number of practical ways to help.

THE IMPACT OF SMOKING ON HEALTHCARE

Currently 28% of men and 26% of women in the UK smoke.[2] Traditionally men have smoked more than women, but now women are catching up. Lifelong smokers have a one in two chance of dying prematurely.[3] Many serious and debilitating diseases can be caused by smoking, the most common being cancer, coronary heart disease and COPD (chronic bronchitis/emphysema).

Smoking places a great burden on the health service. Healthcare costs for smokers at any given age are as much as 40% higher than those for non-smokers. Treating people with smoking-related diseases costs the NHS approximately £1.5 billion per year.[4] Helping people to give up smoking is demonstrably cost-effective.[5] The cost per life-year saved of a fully integrated comprehensive cessation service is about £900, which is much cheaper than other medical interventions.

In 1998 the Government published a White Paper, *Smoking Kills*, and since that time specialist NHS services for smokers have been set up across the UK. Nicotine replacement therapy (NRT) and bupropion hydrochloride (Zyban) are both now available on prescription, and evidence-based guidelines for health professionals have been published.[5] The Department of Health broadcasts an anti-smoking publicity campaign on TV and radio. In February 2003, a ban on all forms of tobacco advertising was introduced in the UK.

THE ROLE OF THE PRACTICE NURSE

All practice nurses see, in their daily work, the health-related consequences of smoking. Your intervention to help a patient quit smoking may be the most important single influence you can have on their health. Stopping smoking is beneficial at any stage in life; it is never too late to stop.[2]

National smoking cessation guidelines for health professionals have been published and confirm that a combination of support and pharmacotherapy is extremely effective, even for those who are highly addicted.[5] These guidelines are known as *The 4 As* (Box 14.1).

The 4 As

Ask

All patients should have their smoking (or other tobacco use) status established and checked at every visit (Box 14.2), and a system should be devised to record this in their notes. The guidelines suggest noting a patient as a non-smoker, recent ex-smoker or smoker and, if currently smoking, whether or not they display any interest in stopping. This can be assessed with an open-ended question such as 'When was the last time you considered stopping smoking?' followed by 'Are you interested in stopping smoking at the moment?'

Advise

Even if they do not currently wish to quit, all smokers should be advised of the value of stopping and the risks to health if they continue to smoke. The advice should be clear, firm and tailored to their personal situation.

Assist

If the smoker would like to stop, help should be offered and the following key points can be covered in 5–10 minutes:

- Set a date to stop – stop completely on that day.
- Review past experience – what helped, what hindered?
- Plan ahead – identify likely problems; make a plan to deal with them.
- Tell family and friends and enlist their support.

BOX 14.1   The 4 As of smoking cessation

ASK: about smoking at every opportunity

ADVISE: all smokers to stop

ASSIST: the smoker to stop

ARRANGE: follow-up

BOX 14.2   Opportunities to discuss smoking in general practice

- New patient bookings
- Well woman/man checks
- Cervical cytology screening
- Patients with asthma, COPD or other smoking-related problems
- When people have coughs, colds or chest infections
- Asthmatic checks on children whose parents smoke
- Diabetes check
- Contraceptive pill check

- Recommend the use of NRT or bupropion to smokers who want to stop, and provide accurate information and advice on both.

Arrange

Depending on your practice facilities, arrange a follow-up visit to the practice specialist and further visits after that if possible. Most smokers make several attempts to stop before finally succeeding (the average is about five to six attempts), and thus relapse is a normal part of the process. If a smoker has made repeated attempts to stop and failed, experienced severe withdrawal symptoms and/or requested more intensive help, it is impor-tant to consider referring them to an NHS specialist service.

When starting a discussion it might be useful to ask the following questions:

- You've told me you are a smoker, what do you enjoy most about smoking?
- How long have you been smoking?
- Have you changed anything about the way you smoke? If so, why?
- Have you ever considered giving up? If so, why?
- Have you tried quitting before? For how long did you stop?
- How did you feel the last time you stopped?
- What was the situation that made you return to smoking?
- Are you planning another attempt in the near future?
- What are the reasons behind your wanting to quit?
- Would you like some information or help from me now?

Use open questions and a facilitative approach to help your clients clarify their relationship to cigarettes. Offer them the NHS booklet *Giving Up for Life*, which includes self-help exercises and practical advice on the process of stopping.

Withdrawal symptoms

Many smokers experience withdrawal symptoms, caused by nicotine leaving the body. These can include craving (an intense desire to smoke that typically lasts 2–3 minutes), increased appetite, light-headed or dizzy feelings (caused by an increase in oxygen levels), a worsened cough, tearfulness, anxiety, irritability, loss of concentration and sleep disturbance.

Such withdrawal symptoms can make it hard for people to stay stopped. It is therefore important to explain that using a course of NRT or bupropion will help reduce the symptoms, increasing their chances of success.

TREATMENTS TO AID SMOKING CESSATION

The National Institute for Health and Clinical Excellence (NICE) has issued guidelines on the use of NRT and bupropion for smoking cessation.[6] The review shows that the main smoking cessation treatments (NRT and bupropion) are among the most cost-effective of all healthcare interventions and, as far as the NHS is concerned, represent extremely good value for money.

Bupropion hydrochloride (Zyban)

Bupropion is an effective non-nicotine treatment that has helped many smokers to stop.[7] A course of tablets lasts 2 months and smokers stop smoking during the second week of the course.

It works by reducing both the desire to smoke and the withdrawal symptoms incurred. It is available only on prescription and is not suitable for everyone, so a full medical history is required before it can be prescribed.

Nicotine replacement therapy

There are several NRT products available, including chewing gum, skin patches, nasal spray, sublingual micro-tabs, lozenges and an inhalator. There is no controlled trial evidence favouring

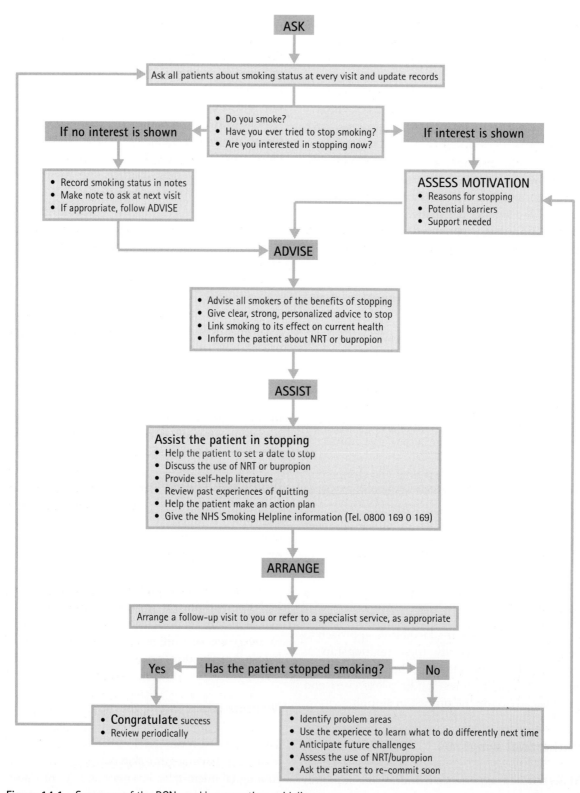

ASK

Ask all patients about smoking status at every visit and update records

- Do you smoke?
- Have you ever tried to stop smoking?
- Are you interested in stopping now?

If no interest is shown

If interest is shown

- Record smoking status in notes
- Make note to ask at next visit
- If appropriate, follow ADVISE

ASSESS MOTIVATION
- Reasons for stopping
- Potential barriers
- Support needed

ADVISE

- Advise all smokers of the benefits of stopping
- Give clear, strong, personalized advice to stop
- Link smoking to its effect on current health
- Inform the patient about NRT or bupropion

ASSIST

Assist the patient in stopping
- Help the patient to set a date to stop
- Discuss the use of NRT or bupropion
- Provide self-help literature
- Review past experiences of quitting
- Help the patient make an action plan
- Give the NHS Smoking Helpline information (Tel. 0800 169 0 169)

ARRANGE

Arrange a follow-up visit to you or refer to a specialist service, as appropriate

Yes   **Has the patient stopped smoking?**   **No**

- **Congratulate** success
- Review periodically

- Identify problem areas
- Use the experiece to learn what to do differently next time
- Anticipate future challenges
- Assess the use of NRT/bupropion
- Ask the patient to re-commit soon

Figure 14.1   Summary of the RCN smoking cessation guidelines.

any one of these products over another. A course of treatment usually lasts 10–12 weeks and is available on general sale, via NHS prescription or in a pharmacy.

Unlike tobacco smoke NRT does not contain tar and carbon monoxide and there is no evidence to suggest that nicotine alone causes cancer. NRT usually provides nicotine in a way that is slower and less satisfying, but safer and less addictive than cigarettes.

Clinical trials have shown that NRT doubles the chance of success for smokers wishing to stop. Using NRT allows the smoker to concentrate on breaking the social and psychological habits while also controlling the physical cravings.

SUPPORTING SMOKERS TO QUIT

It can be frustrating working with smokers if you expect them all to stop. Prochaska and Di Clemente's stages-of-change model[10] describes a series of five predictable stages that a smoker endures. It demonstrates that stopping smoking is more of a process than a single event.[8] The stages are:

- *Pre-contemplation stage – contented smokers*:
  - no interest at all in changing behaviour
  - many personal advantages to the habit.
- *Contemplation stage – considering changing*:
  - thinking about changing
  - acknowledging some dangers and risks
  - still have reasons for continuing.
- *Preparation stage*:
  - realizing that stopping is beneficial
  - believing stopping is possible
  - making plans to stop.
- *Action stage*:
  - changing behaviour
  - actually stopping.
- *Maintenance*:
  - staying stopped
  - coping without relapse
  - managing temptation.
- *Relapse*:
  - returning to smoking.

From this model it is clear that a smoker needs to consider stopping, understand the dangers, apply the risks and realize that stopping is beneficial. Practice nurses can help people go through this process by linking poor health to their smoking. You will be aware when an illness is diagnosed or deterioration found. You will meet heavy smokers with chest infections, chart a decreasing lung function and observe reducing mobility.

Even when a patient is not interested in stopping smoking, it is helpful to give them clear advice relating to the risks of smoking and the benefits of stopping. Tell them about the support available should they consider stopping in the future.

Stopping smoking can be quite easy for some smokers and an enormous task for others. The smoker is the expert on themselves and their habit. When trying to give up, the smoker may just want to talk to a sensitive listener about their difficulties and achievements.

SUMMARY

Smoking is classified as a chronic relapsing condition. Staying stopped takes practice and determination. Each smoker needs time and support to realize the risks of continuing and the

---

ESSENTIAL SKILLS

- Understand the impact of tobacco as the lead cause of disability and premature death in the UK
- Knowledge and ability to apply the National Smoking Cessation Guidelines (the 4 As)
- Understand the effectiveness of pharmacotherapy in smoking cessation
- Be familiar with the NHS smoking cessation services, and know how to refer smokers to them
- Know which NHS materials are appropriate to use

benefits of quitting. Helping someone to stop smoking is not about giving advice; it is about asking the right questions. It is usual for people to make five or six attempts to quit. The practice nurse's role is to work in partnership with the smoker as he or she goes through this process.

REFERENCES

1. Callum C. The UK Smoking Epidemic: Deaths in 1995. London: Health Education Authority, 1998.
2. National Statistics. Living in Britain: Results from the 2001 General Household Survey. London: National Statistics, 2002. Available at: http://www.statistics.gov.uk/lib
3. Doll R, Peto R, Wheatley K, Gray R, Sutherland I. Mortality in relation to smoking: 40 years' observations on male British doctors. BMJ 1994; 309: 901–911.
4. Buck D, Godfrey C. Helping Smokers Give Up: Guidance for Purchasers on Cost Effectiveness. London: Health Education Authority, 1994.
5. Parrott S, Godfrey C, Raw M, West R, McNeill A. Guidance for commissioners on the cost effectiveness of smoking cessation interventions. Thorax 1998; 53(Suppl 5, Pt 2): 1–38.
6. Department of Health. Smoking Kills: A White Paper on Tobacco Presented to Parliament by the Secretary of State for Health. London: The Stationery Office, 1998.
7. West R, McNeill A, Raw M. Smoking cessation guidelines for health professionals: an update. Thorax 2000; **55**: 987–999.
8. NICE. Guidance on the use of nicotine replacement therapy (NRT) and bupropion for smoking cessation. London: NICE, 2002. Available at: http://www.nice.org.uk
9. Jorenby DE, Leischow SJ, Nides MA, et al. A controlled trial of sustained-release bupropion, a nicotine patch, or both for smoking cessation. N Engl J Med 1999; 340: 685–691.
10. Prochaska J, DiClemente C. Stages and processes of self change in smoking: towards an integrative model of change. J Consult Clin Psychol 1983; 51: 390–395.
11. Department of Health. Statistics on Smoking Cessation Services in England: April 2000 to March 2001. Department of Health Statistical Bulletin 2001/32. London: DoH, 2001.

FURTHER INFORMATION

NHS Smoking Cessation Services have now been set up within each health authority. They provide specialist support to smokers through clinics, group work or one-to-one sessions. Their work is extremely effective, and with the help of these services around 132,500 people set a quit date during 2000–2001.[11]

NHS Smoking Helpline (Tel. 0800 169 0169) offers support to people who wish to give up smoking, which they back up with a range of useful leaflets and literature. The lines are generally open between 9 a.m. and 5 p.m., Monday to Friday. Health professionals can order free NHS resources and a professional support pack to aid their work.

Royal College of Nursing (RCN) runs a Tobacco Education Project that aims to increase members' knowledge and skills when working with smokers. The project runs training programmes, seminars and conferences for nurses. For more information contact: Jennifer Percival, RCN Tobacco Education Project Manager, PO Box 78, Kings Langley WD4 8ZB (Tel. 01442 240728). The RCN publication *Clearing the Air 2: Smoking and Tobacco Control – An Updated Guide for Nurses* is available from RCN Direct (Tel. 0845 772 6100).

Chapter 15

Nutrition

Jane DeVille-Almond

Nutrition is probably the one area of health that all primary care nurses have to deal with at some time. It is a topic relevant to patients in all age groups, from small babies to the elderly, and encompasses a whole range of issues, such as: what milks to recommend for babies; teenagers and eating disorders; specific health conditions that require a special diet; obesity in all age groups; right through to concerns with the elderly, malnutrition and bowel disorders. In the NHS Plan, the NHS Cancer Plan and the National Service Frameworks for Coronary Heart Disease, Diabetes and Older People, diet and nutrition are highlighted as key areas for action.[1-5]

Our daily diet is the key to maintaining and regaining good health, and the practice nurse needs a basic understanding of nutritional requirements. The diet needs to provide sufficient:

- water
- protein for tissue repair, maintenance and growth
- carbohydrate and fat for energy
- vitamins and minerals for the regulation of physiological processes.

No type of food contains all the necessary nutrients, so patients should be encouraged to eat a variety of foods from each food group, in the proportions shown in Box 15.1.[6]

BOX 15.1   The cornerstones of sound diet and nutrition

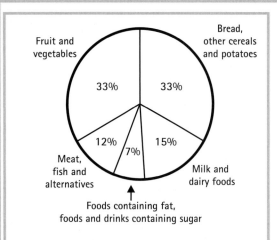

The subdivisions of the pie chart illustrate the basic rules for a healthy diet.

In response to the increasing prevalence of obesity, a recent Government White Paper on public health, *Choosing Health*,[7] is proposing a traffic-light system of food labelling to help people make wise choices:

- **Green–light foods**: fruit and vegetables – eat at least five portions a day
- **Orange–light foods**: eggs, cheese, fish, meat, bread, pasta and rice – eat in moderate amounts
- **Red–light foods**: foods high in fat, sugar and salt, such as cakes, biscuits, fatty meats, fried food, snack foods, chocolates and soft drinks – eat with caution and do not let them make up the bulk of any diet

- Select a variety of foods from each group in the proportion shown
- Eat at least 5 portions of fruit and vegetables a day
- Eat foods containing fats and sugars sparingly and select lower fat options where possible
- Use less salt
- Drink plenty of fluid: 6 to 10 cups or glasses a day

FRUIT AND VEGETABLES: WHY FIVE A DAY?

It has been estimated that diet might contribute to the development of one-third of all cancers and that, after reducing smoking, increasing fruit and vegetable intake is the second most important cancer-prevention strategy.[2] Fruit and vegetables are good sources of the antioxidant vitamins A, C and E (Box 15.2) that play a major part in protecting against the development of coronary heart disease, stroke and some cancers, and many are also naturally high in folic acid, potassium and fibre. Higher consumption can also help lower blood pressure, delay the development of cataracts, reduce the symptoms of asthma, improve bowel function and help in managing diabetes.[8]

Fruit and vegetable consumption is, on average, low among the population in England (less than three portions a day), and according to

BOX 15.2   Sources of the antioxidant (ACE) vitamins

- **Vitamin A**: especially high levels in dark green vegetables, carrots and red peppers
- **Vitamin C**: in many fruits, with especially high levels in blackcurrants, strawberries, raspberries, oranges, kiwi fruit and mangoes
- **Vitamin E**: in leafy vegetables, vegetable oils, plums and nuts
- Tomatoes are an excellent source of all the ACE vitamins and also contain lycopene, another potent antioxidant
- Wholegrain cereals, nuts and seeds are also good sources

recent press reports has dropped to two since the Government launched its '5 a day' campaign. So what may prevent people eating more fruit? Poor access to and availability of good quality, affordable fruit and vegetables may be a factor for some, but for many it may be down to attitudes and awareness, and this is where the practice nurse can have most influence (Box 15.3). It is important for practice nurses to find out what is happening in their area, such as healthy eating initiatives in schools and other partnership programmes, and work with other healthcare professionals and agencies.

CARBOHYDRATES

Carbohydrates are the body's preferred energy source, which is why athletes consume large amounts to help them maintain their energy levels. They can be refined or unrefined, and 'complex' or 'simple' in their chemical structure.

BOX 15.3   Tips on implementing '5 portions a day' of fruit and vegetables[8]

- A portion is roughly 80 g (about 3 oz)
- These portions can be fresh, frozen, canned or dried
- A portion of dried fruit is about the same as you would eat if it were fresh (e.g. three apricots, two figs)
- Juice can count as only one portion a day, however much you drink, and must be fresh squeezed, not from concentrate. Also note that many fruit juices are high in sugar
- Beans and other pulses (kidney beans, lentils, chickpeas) can only count once a day, however much you eat, as they contain fibre but not the same mixture of vitamins, minerals and other nutrients as fruit and vegetables
- Potatoes do not count towards '5 a day' portions because, like rice, pasta and bread, they are considered a 'starchy' food. However, starch foods are still an important part of a balanced diet

---

Starchy carbohydrates are foods such as bread, cereals, rice, pasta and potatoes. Grains and food made from them can be unrefined (wholegrain rice, wholemeal bread, porridge oats and wholewheat pasta) or refined (white rice, white bread and pasta made from white flour), the latter being foods from which the high-fibre parts of the grain (the bran and the germ) have been removed.

Starch is a complex carbohydrate, in which simple sugars are bonded together into long chains, or polysaccharides. Because these chains have to be broken down by digestive enzymes into individual glucose molecules before they can be absorbed, the energy in complex carbohydrates is released relatively slowly. Fibre, a non-starch polysaccharide that is plentiful in unrefined carbohydrates, fruit and vegetables, is not digested but is nevertheless an important part of the diet.

Simple carbohydrates are smaller sugar molecules that can be digested to glucose and absorbed much more quickly than complex carbohydrates. They are a more immediate source of energy but their rapid absorption increases the chance of the body converting excess energy to fat if an excess of sugar is absorbed. Glucose is the main sugar in many foods, but others include sucrose (table sugar), fructose in fruit, lactose in milk, and galactose in milk and yoghurt. Foods such as cakes, pastries, biscuits, chocolate, jam, honey, soft drinks, tinned-fruit syrup, chutney and some puddings are high in simple carbohydrates, which represent 'empty' calories. Many processed foods have hidden sugars, and patients should be encouraged to read the packaging labels.

FATS IN THE DIET

Fats make food taste good and are an essential component in a balanced diet – they carry and aid in the absorption of the fat-soluble vitamins A, D, E and K, and provide essential fatty acids, such as linoleic and linolenic acids, necessary for proper growth.

However, as they are high in calories (they are the most concentrated source of dietary energy) and contain few nutrients they should form only a small part of a healthy diet. The two main types of dietary fats – saturated fats and unsaturated fats – have different effects on cholesterol levels.

Saturated fats

Saturated fats are the type we should try particularly to restrict in the diet, because they raise levels of total cholesterol and artery-clogging low-density lipid (LDL) cholesterol. Eating too much of them increases the risk of heart disease. They come mainly from animal sources (e.g. the fat on red meat and under the skin of poultry), but also occur in some vegetable oils such as coconut oil and palm oil. They are usually hard at room temperature – just look at a cold frying pan after cooking sausage or bacon – and are found in cooking fats such as lard and full-fat dairy products (butter, cheese, whole milk).

Also best avoided are trans-unsaturated fats, which are formed during the hardening of vegetable oils by a process called partial hydrogenation and found in hard margarines. These not only raise LDL cholesterol but also lower levels of beneficial high-density lipid (HDL) cholesterol.

Like simple carbohydrates, saturated and trans-unsaturated fats are often 'hidden' in processed foods such as cakes, biscuits, chocolate and puddings. When checking food labels, patients should look out for both saturated fat and hydrogenated vegetable oils/fats.

Unsaturated fats

Unsaturated fats are essential to the body, although only in small amounts. Mostly of plant origin, they are usually liquid at room temperature and may be polyunsaturated or monounsaturated.

Polyunsaturated fats lower the levels of LDL cholesterol, but also those of protective HDL cholesterol. They are found in vegetable oils such as sunflower, corn and soya oils, many low-fat spreads and oily fish such as salmon, mackerel, pilchards and sardines.

Monounsaturated fats lower levels of LDL cholesterol, but not those of HDL cholesterol. They are found in olive, rapeseed (canola) and ground-nut oils and a wide range of low-fat spreads.

Omega–3 fats

The message to cut down on saturated fat and swap to unsaturated oils and spreads has been part of dietary advice for many years, and consumers and food manufacturers have responded. However, this shift in the balance of fats consumed has resulted in a relative lack in the diet of the polyunsaturated fats known as the omega-3s. Omega-3 fatty acids are beneficial for the primary prevention of heart disease and, after a myocardial infarction, reduce the risk of a further cardiac event.[9, 10] They reduce blood triglyceride levels, help prevent thrombosis and reduce blood pressure, and reduce the risk of arrhythmia. There is also mounting evidence that these fats are important for other reasons. They are known to be important in brain development in fetal life and during infancy, and have been found to help inflammatory conditions such as rheumatoid arthritis and asthma, to improve forced expiratory volume in people with cystic fibrosis and to be of benefit in depression and Alzheimer's disease.

Although omega-3 fatty acids can be made in the body from the essential fatty acid linolenic acid, good sources of which are rapeseed oil, soya oil and walnuts, a major source is oily fish. Weekly consumption of oily fish should be encouraged.[11] Tinned mackerel, sardines and salmon are easy to store and make a quick meal, but advise patients not to buy fish tinned in oil or mayonnaise.

All polyunsaturated fats, including the omega-3s, are increasingly recognized as important to human health. However, all fats contain the same number of calories, so in terms of weight control we should be limiting our intake of fat, no matter which type it may be.

VITAMINS

There are two main groups of vitamins, fat soluble and water soluble. Fat-soluble vitamins (A, D and E) can be found in foods such as fish, meat, butter, milk and plant oils. They can be stored in the liver and adipose tissue, so toxic levels can accumulate with excess intake. Water-soluble vitamins (the B vitamins, vitamin C and folic acid) are easily lost from foods and the body, so it is difficult to overdose on them. It is these in which deficiency is most likely.

MINERALS

Various minerals are essential for a healthy body; those of particular nutritional significance include iron, iodine and zinc. Iodine deficiency is often characterized by marked enlargement of the thyroid gland and may occur in areas where water and soil are deficient in iodine.

Zinc is particularly important in periods of growth and during wound healing; animal products are the main source.

Iron's main function is as a component of haemoglobin, but it is also important in many enzyme processes and in the immune response. Small amounts are lost from the body, mainly through the gastrointestinal tract in blood, desquamated cells and bile, and menstruation may also add to variable losses. The most nutritionally effective iron is found in meat, so some vegetarians may require supplements.[12]

SALT

There is thought to be a link between salt consumption and hypertension, but the exact connection is not understood. Most people today eat far more salt than the daily 1 g (about one-fifth of a teaspoonful) the body needs. The recommended maximum is 6 g a day. It is the sodium content of salt that contributes to high blood pressure, and on food labels salt appears as sodium, 2.5 g of sodium being equivalent to 6 g of salt.

To help patients cut down on salt, first advise them to try not adding salt to their food at the table. Later, they should try cooking without adding salt, using herbs and spices to add flavour instead. Most people find that within a month or so their palate will have adjusted so that they no longer like salty foods.

WEIGHT CONTROL

Food energy is measured in calories. If we eat more energy than our body needs it is stored as fat and we put on weight. Energy requirements vary according to a person's weight, age, sex and levels of activity, but women should aim to take in 1,500–2,000 calories a day, while men, being more muscular, need around 2,000–2,500 calories per day in caloric intake. Most people will burn at least 80 calories an hour, even if they stay in bed all day.

If you wish to lose weight, try decreasing your daily calorie intake by about 500 calories. One kilogram of fat has 7,000 calories, so this should see you lose about 0.5–1.0 kg a week (never aim for more). If you fail to lose weight after a few weeks, then cut your daily intake by another 500 calories, and remember it is also important to take regular exercise. Daily intake should never be reduced by more than 1,000 calories except under the supervision of a doctor or dietitian.

Many people think they burn up more calories than they really do (Box 15.4). Most packaged foods have calorie content per 100 g printed on the label, although from this it can be difficult to work out the calories per portion. Several good calorie-conversion books are available and every surgery should have at least one to refer to (see Further Reading at the end of this chapter).

BOX 15.4   Exercise and burning up calories

- To burn up 100 calories, a person needs to walk at a moderate pace for 30 minutes
- If you exceed your daily calorie requirements by eating a small bar of chocolate (around 250 calories), you need to walk for at least 75 minutes to burn it off
- Adults are advised to take at least 30 minutes of moderate exercise on at least 5 days a week
- Children should have at least an hour of exercise every day

---

BOX 15.5   Obesity in the UK

- 1 in 2 people is overweight or obese
- About 1 in 5 people is clinically obese (BMI > 30)
- By 2010 around 25% of the population (1 in 4) will be clinically obese
- Around 52,500 lives are lost each year because of weight-related illnesses
- Obesity costs the NHS about £7.5 billion a year, one of the largest expenditures for healthcare services

---

Obesity

Being overweight is likely to knock 9 years off your life expectancy, and obese patients are far more likely to develop hypertension, diabetes, arthritis, joint problems, heart disease, strokes, respiratory disorders and some cancers. So the steady increase in the prevalence of obesity is one of the most serious health issues in modern society (Box 15.5).

In Britain, the past 60 years have seen eating habits change considerably. In 1940, for example, the average diet contained 31% fat and 53% carbohydrate; by 1990 the balance had shifted to 43% fat (up 12%) and 45% carbohydrate (down 8%).[13] It is this change in diet, together with increasingly sedentary jobs and lifestyles, that has had a massive effect on the population's weight.[14]

All patients attending the surgery should have a body mass index (BMI) and waist measurement recorded fairly regularly (at least once a year), especially if at risk from weight gain or other related diseases, and any unhealthy weight gain or loss should be discussed. A calculator (or special BMI wheel) is useful to work out BMIs (Box 15.6). Waist measurement is important because central abdominal fat, as seen in people with apple-shaped bodies, is particularly associated with health problems such as type 2 diabetes and heart disease. Weight carried on the hips is less of a health risk, and a 'pear shape' is much more common in women.

Overweight and obese patients losing 5–10% of their body weight will have substantial health benefits. Patients should be encouraged to lose around 1 kg (or 2 lb) per week as, unlike a crash diet, slow and steady weight loss will often result in long-term success.

The Government is considering offering health coaches and weight-watcher classes on prescription, to help combat the rising levels of obesity. In some cases, GPs may prescribe one of the drugs shown to have some positive effect in weight control; patients taking them will require regular monitoring. Sibutramine (Reductil) works by boosting the signal to stop eating so that patients feel fuller sooner and eat less, and orlistat (Xenical) blocks the digestion of fat.

Morbidly obese patients may be referred for bariatric surgery, in which stomach size, and hence food intake, is reduced by surgically placing an adjustable band around the stomach.

IS THERE A NEED FOR VITAMIN SUPPLEMENTS?

A normal balanced diet should provide an adequate supply of all the nutrients, and important non-nutrients such as fibre, necessary to maintain

---

BOX 15.6   Monitoring patients' body mass index and waist measurement

BMI = weight (kg) ÷ height^2 (m^2)
BMI < 18 = underweight
Patients who are underweight (especially if weight loss has been sudden) should be monitored and referred to the GP if you are worried. Being underweight may lead to health problems, such as amenorrhoea, infertility and osteoporosis, and weight loss can be an indicator of problems such as malabsorption, anorexia, other eating disorders and bowel cancer

BMI 18–24.9 = normal
Advise the patient to maintain their weight around the current level

BMI 25–30 = overweight
Advise the patient to lose weight, especially if there are other health risks such as diabetes, heart disease, hypertension or a family history of obesity

BMI > 30 = obese
BMI > 40 = morbidly obese
Encourage the patient to lose weight and give extra support. If obesity is ignored it is likely to lead to health problems. Monitoring may include regular weighing and the opportunity to discuss healthy eating or referral to the GP for further help

Waist measurement
A measurement of > 37 inches for women or > 40 inches for men puts health at risk

---

a healthy body. There are times when vitamin supplements may be of benefit, such as during pregnancy or severe illness, but they should be taken as recommended by the GP as some vitamins (e.g. vitamin A) are toxic in high doses.

Strict vegetarians (vegans) who avoid dairy products may have to rely on supplements and their diet often lacks vitamin B$_{12}$. The vegetarian diet is also high in water-absorbing fibre, so it is important to remind vegetarians to drink plenty of fluid.[12]

WHAT ABOUT SPECIAL DIETS?

Weight reduction

No faddy diets should be encouraged, but many patients will insist on trying them to give them a kick-start into losing weight. Practice nurses need to support patients in whatever diet they choose, but gently encourage them to work towards making long-term changes in eating habits that they will be able to maintain.

When slimming diets such as the Atkins diet hit the headlines, patients want to know if they work. Most diets do work in the short term, especially if followed strictly to the letter. However, when patients revert to their previous eating pattern after successful weight loss on a 'diet', they will usually not only regain the lost weight but also put on more.

Many commercial weight-management clinics have high success rates, often because of the extra support they provide, and there is no reason why a patient cannot also be supported by the practice nurse. It is worth knowing which weight-management clinics are run in your area. This information can often be obtained from your patients.

Diabetes

People with diabetes need to control their blood sugar. However, there are no foods that they should never eat, and neither Diabetes UK nor the Food Standards Agency recommend the purchase of special 'diabetic' foods. In their view these are expensive and not necessarily healthier or more suitable for people with diabetes than other foods. People with diabetes should try to maintain a healthy weight and eat a diet that is:

- low in fat (particularly saturated fat)
- low in sugar
- low in salt
- high in fruit and vegetables (at least five portions a day)
- high in starchy carbohydrate foods, such as bread, chapattis, rice, pasta and yams, which should form the basis of meals.

Coeliac disease

Patients with coeliac disease should stick to a strict gluten-free diet; otherwise the general dietary advice is as for any patient. Wheat flour is the main source of gluten, and Coeliac UK produces a guide to gluten-free foods and other useful dietary information. Most patients diagnosed with coeliac disease will know what they can and cannot eat.

Malnutrition

Groups that may be at particular risk of undernourishment include the homeless, the elderly (especially those who have recently been in hospital or live alone), alcoholics and those with behavioural disturbances, including mental illness and eating disorders such as anorexia nervosa or bulimia. A special eye should also be kept on some children, particularly those whom you may consider vulnerable. If a patient is severely underweight it is important to investigate the problem. Undernourishment is often associated with chronic disease, and when a patient is unwell adequate levels of protein, carbohydrate, certain fats, iron and zinc in the diet may be of particular significance in maintaining the body's immunological functions.[12]

CONCLUSION

It is important for the practice nurse to recognize the key role of healthy eating in protecting and improving the health of patients. The importance of what we eat is highlighted more than ever by the global increase in the prevalence of heart disease, stroke, cancer, obesity and type 2 diabetes.

Energy-rich diets that are high in fat and sodium and low in fibre and fruit and vegetables play a central part in the development of disease risk factors such as hyperlipidaemia, hypertension, insulin resistance and atherogenesis, and these risk factors can be reduced if individuals adopt a healthier way of eating.

ESSENTIAL SKILLS

- Understanding basic nutritional needs
- Advising patients on what is a healthy diet
- Explaining why the Government recommends we eat '5 a day'
- Understanding the long-term health consequences of obesity
- Helping people understand the link between calorie intake and exercise and weight control
- Advising on special diets

REFERENCES

1. Department of Health. The NHS Plan. A Plan for Investment, a Plan for Reform. London: The Stationery Office; 2000. Available at: http://www.publications.doh.gov.uk/nhsplan/nhsplan.htm

2. Department of Health. NHS Cancer Plan. London: DoH, 2000.

3. Department of Health. National Service Framework for Coronary Heart Disease. London: DoH, 2000.

4. Department of Health. National Service Framework for Older People. London: DoH, 2001. Available at: http://www.dh.gov.uk

5. Department of Health. National Service Framework for Diabetes: Standards. London: DoH; 2001. Available at: http://www.dh.gov.uk/nsf/diabetes.htm

6. British Meat Nutrition Education Service. Enjoying a Healthy Diet is all about Getting the Balance Right. February 2003. Available at: http://www.bmesonline.org.uk/pdf/gettingthebalanceright.pdf

7. Department of Health. Choosing Health: Making Healthier Choices Easier. Public Health White Paper CM 6374. London: DoH, 2004.

8. Department of Health. 5 A DAY: Health Benefits. Just Eat More (Fruit and Vegetables). London: DoH, 2003. Available at: http://www.5aday.nhs.uk

9. British Nutrition Foundation. n-3 Fatty Acids and Health [briefing paper]. London: BNF, 1999.

10. GISSI-Prevenzione. Dietary supplementation with n-3 polyunsaturated fatty acids and vitamin E after myocardial infarction. Lancet 1999; 354: 447–455.

11. Committee on Medical Aspects of Food and Nutrition Policy (COMA). Nutritional Aspects of Cardiovascular Disease. London: DoH, 1994.

12. Alexander M, Fawcett J, Runciman P. Nursing Practice: Hospitals and Home. London: Harcourt; 2000.

13. National Audit Office. Tackling Obesity in England. London: The Stationery Office; 2001. Available at: http://www.nao.org.uk/publications/nao_reports/00–01/0001220.pdf

14. DEFRA. National Food Survey 1998. London: The Stationery Office; 1999. National Food Survey datasets available at: http://statistics.defra.gov.uk/esg/publications/nfs/default.asp

FURTHER READING

Sims J, Walton T. The Calorie Carb and Fat Bible. Peterborough: Weight Loss Resources, 2004.

USEFUL WEBSITES

National Obesity Forum: http://www.nationalobesityforum.org.uk

Diabetes UK: http://www.diabetesuk.org.uk

British Heart Foundation: http://www.bhf.org.uk

Coeliac UK, the charity supporting people with gluten intolerance: http://www.coeliacuk.org.uk

British Meat Education Service: http://www.bmesonline.org.uk

Chapter 16

Obesity

Nerys Williams

More than half of all UK adults are now overweight.[1] Helping your patients to achieve a healthy lifestyle has never been more important. According to a recent report by the World Health Organization, we are in the grips of an obesity epidemic.[2] Obesity is a key risk factor in the development of many conditions, including type 2 diabetes, cardiovascular disease, hypertension and stroke, and is associated with an increased risk of cancers.[2]

Obesity is defined according to the body mass index (BMI): the ratio of weight (in kilograms) divided by height (in metres) squared. Levels below 25 kg/m² are considered normal, overweight is defined as having a BMI between 25 and 30, obesity as having a BMI over 30 and morbid obesity as having a BMI over 40.

However, these figures apply to European populations. Because Asian populations have comorbidities at lower BMIs than the corresponding white population, it has been suggested that in Asian populations a BMI above 23 should indicate overweight and one above 25 indicate obesity.[3]

BMI also has drawbacks for measuring obesity in children and the elderly and, while it allows for the influence of height on obesity, high BMIs occur in elite athletes, whose heavy muscle bulk weighs more than fat. BMI is not the 'one size fits all' measure as far as obesity is concerned, and its limitations need to be recognized. Yet BMI remains important, as it is often used in research as an indicator of the risks and success of treatment.

The amount of body fat is not the only important factor, but also where it is located. Central, or apple-shaped, obesity, with a waist circumference of > 102 cm in men and > 88 cm in women (or > 90 cm for men and > 80 cm for women of South Asian origin), is strongly associated with an increased risk of metabolic syndrome (hypertension, diabetes and abnormal lipids) when compared with normal weight and waist circumference.[4]

PREVALENCE

The current prevalence of obesity is between 14% and 20% in industrial countries,[2] but the fastest increases, particularly in childhood obesity, are seen in developing countries such as China. In the UK, data from the Health Survey of England and Wales revealed an increase in the prevalence of obesity from 6% and 8% for women and men, respectively, in 1980, to 8% and 12% in 1990, and to over 21% for both sexes in the year 2000. The situation is now so advanced that more than 50% of adults are overweight.[1]

The reasons for this rise in the incidence of obesity are complex. There is a genetic predisposition to obesity, which may explain up to 30–50% of its heritability.[5, 6] However, the gene pool has not changed rapidly enough over the last 10–15 years to account for the steep increase in the numbers of people affected by excessive weight. Changes in lifestyle affecting both energy intake and energy expenditure have played an important part.

FOOD AND ACTIVITY: THE ENERGY BALANCE

Increased calorie intake

Food is now cheaper, more easily available and packed with calories through increased amounts of fat, refined sugars and less complex carbohydrates. Consumption of alcohol, a potent yet often silent source of calories, has also increased in both men and women.

Eating patterns have changed, with more snacks, fewer family meals, more eating out and increased portion sizes. Children have greater autonomy in selecting their food and greater spending power, and are influenced by advertising and peer pressure.

Decreased activity

On the activity side of the equation, changes in the way we live have meant that we all use our cars more often, even for short journeys. Children no longer play outside because of perceived dangers. They are driven rather than walk to school, and physical education no longer forms part of every curriculum.

The rise of computer games and the internet have increased the amount of sedentary leisure time, and the increase in labour-saving devices in the home means that housework expends fewer calories as well.

The workplace has changed, with fewer manufacturing and physical jobs and more service-based industries and sedentary work. People spend more time sitting, for example in offices and call centres, and even the energy expended in getting to work has been reduced by locating car parks close to workplace entrances.

HEALTH RISKS

So why should we be concerned by this increase in obesity? The health risks of being overweight have been well defined. For even a moderately raised BMI of between 27 and 30 the risk of breast cancer is increased by 1.3, that of gallstones by 2.7, cancer of the colon by 1.5 and cancer of the pancreas by 1.6, when compared with someone with a normal BMI.[1]

Obesity also has a major effect on the cardiovascular system, and again the relative risk of a raised BMI of between 27 and 30 increases the risk of hypertension by 2.9, heart disease by 2.5 and stroke by 1.6.[1]

One of the most dramatic impacts of the rise in obesity has been the mirrored rise in the incidence of type 2 diabetes. This is not really surprising, as obesity is the main cause of type 2 diabetes, and is fuelling that particular epidemic.

TREATMENT

There is often a discrepancy between patients' goals and those of their medical professionals. Patients often want to lose large amounts of weight, and so set themselves highly ambitious targets and fail to meet them. From a medical point of view, many health benefits can be obtained by a reduction of 5–10% of body weight.

Lifestyle modification remains a cornerstone of obesity treatment, with a concentration on dietary adjustment and increased activity, but additional help is now available in the form of medication and surgery.

Dietary management

Current dietary management focuses on healthy eating principles and adopting a fixed calorie diet approximately 600 calories below that required to maintain a constant weight. If complied with, such diets can reliably lead to loss of 1–1.5 lb per week.

Other advice includes a daily intake of five portions of fruit and vegetables, three meals per day, no snacking between meals, and restricting alcohol intake, as this is often an invisible source of calories.

A switch to low-fat foods, even without restricting the amount of food eaten, often results in weight loss.

The importance of activity

Increased levels of activity should be encouraged, as this not only provides individuals with cardiovascular benefits but also aids weight loss. While exercise by itself only confers a modest weight loss, it has been proven to be valuable in keeping weight off.

For very obese individuals, simple techniques, such as walking rather than using the lift at work, using stairs rather than elevators and trying to get off a bus one stop earlier, can all assist in burning off calories. For those patients who have done little exercise in the recent past the prospect of the gym may deter them from making changes. The key message is that it is activity that is important, not just exercise.

Drug management

There are two drugs commonly licensed for use in the UK. Orlistat (Xenical) is a pancreatic and gastric lipase inhibitor, which reduces the amount of fat absorbed into the body. It is taken three times per day. One of the side-effects is diarrhoea, which is particularly likely if fat is consumed, so patients have to be careful. Orlistat must be used in conjunction with a low-fat, healthy diet and increased activity. Only 2% of the drug is absorbed into the body; it brings about weight loss through reducing the calories entering the body from fat eaten in the diet.

The second drug that may be prescribed for obesity is sibutramine (Reductil). Sibutramine is a satiety enhancer, not an appetite suppressant. It has noradrenergic effects that make the patient feel fuller after a smaller portion of food. Sibutramine is contraindicated in the presence of depression and hypertension; in the early stages of treatment both heart rate and blood pressure need to be measured frequently. The drug works by altering the feeling of fullness, and so reducing the amount of food that is eaten. It is suitable for patients who have particular difficulties with the size of the portions they eat as it aims to retrain the appetite to be satisfied with less. It can be continued for a maximum of 12 months, provided patients meet certain goals for weight loss.

Both orlistat and sibutramine have been recommended by the National Institute for Health and Clinical Excellence (NICE) for use in obese patients, and those who are less overweight but who have coexisting disease.[7, 8] Studies have shown that these medications can help patients to achieve 10% weight loss that can be maintained for 2 years. Maximum benefit is gained by 6 months after therapy is started. Patients who successfully lose weight not only become more mobile but also show improvements in metabolic factors, such as blood glucose and blood pressure. The two medications should not be used together.

Surgery

In a small group of individuals for whom medical treatment is not successful, surgery may be indicated. There are two types of operation: one that restricts food consumption by making the stomach smaller (banding) and one that produces malabsorption by bypassing parts of the digestive tract (biliary–pancreatic bypass). NICE has reviewed the indications for surgery, and published guidance on its use.[9]

MANAGEMENT IN GENERAL PRACTICE

First and foremost, individuals need to be motivated to lose weight, and assisted by an enthusiastic practitioner. There is no magic bullet, and weight loss requires effort and commitment by the patient. Positive motivational techniques need to be employed to highlight the benefits of weight loss and the disadvantages of weight gain.

Interested practice nurses can set up weight-management clinics within primary care, provided they have the skills to motivate and the knowledge to advise on the basic principles of healthy eating. Patients referred to such a clinic would benefit

from having basic measurements of height, weight, BMI, waist circumference, blood pressure and urine analysis taken. Where appropriate and clinically indicated, thyroid function tests should be performed, and Cushing's syndrome should be considered in any centrally obese, hypertensive patient with hirsutism.

During the first consultation it is essential that the practitioner and patient develop a contract. Neither doctors nor nurses should allow themselves to be thought of as the people who provide a magical weight-loss solution. The work is done by the patient, and he or she needs to understand this. The patient also needs to agree to attend the clinic for follow-up, and to establish achievable goals.

Attendance should not, in my opinion, be open-ended. Setting a 3–4 month course at the outset is realistic in terms of expecting to see some benefits. If weight loss does not occur over this period it may not be the right time for the patient to commit. They may need more time and a review later on.

Weight-loss targets are important, and should be staggered to help monitor gradual progress. At each consultation, weight, BMI and waist circumference should be measured. It may be possible to provide encouragement that progress is being made, even if there is no weight loss, if the waist size has been reduced. Studies suggest that frequent support in the early phase of weight loss is more successful than long periods between consultations.

Food and activity diaries can be discussed at each consultation, and further support is available from the pharmaceutical companies, in the form

> ### ESSENTIAL SKILLS
>
> - Ability to assess patients' readiness to lose weight
> - Ability to motivate patients
> - Ability to identify and agree achievable goals
> - To be conversant with current obesity management goal-setting and advice

of nurse support helplines, if medication is prescribed. Treating patients with obesity can be rewarding, and can make a real difference to improving their health and quality of life.

REFERENCES

1. Finer N. Obesity. Clin Med 2003; 3(1): 24.
2. World Health Organization. Obesity: Preventing and Managing the Global Epidemic. Report of a WHO Consultation on Obesity. WHO/ NUT/NCD/981. Geneva: WHO, 1998, pp1–275.
3. Inoue S, Zimmett P. The Asia-Pacific Perspective: Redefining Obesity and its Treatment. Australia: Health Communications, 2000.
4. Han TS, Van Leer EM, Seidell JC, et al. Waist circumference action levels in the identification of cardiovascular risk factors – prevalence study in random sample. BMJ 1995; 311: 1401–1405.
5. Stunkard AJ, Sorenson TI, Hanis C, Teasdale TW, et al. An adoption study of human obesity. N Engl J Med 1986; 314: 193–198.
6. Sorenson TI, Price RA, Stunkard AJ, et al. Genetics of obesity in adult adoptees and their biological siblings. BMJ 1986; 298: 87–90.
7. National Institute for Health and Clinical Excellence. Guidance on the Use of Orlistat for the Treatment of Obesity in Adults. Technology Appraisal Guidance No. 22. London: NICE, 2001.
8. National Institute for Health and Clinical Excellence. Guidance on the Use of Sibutramine for the Treatment of Obesity in Adults. Technology Appraisal Guidance No. 31. London: NICE, 2001.
9. National Institute for Health and Clinical Excellence. Guidance on the Use of Surgery to Aid Weight Reduction for People with Morbid Obesity. Technology Appraisal Guidance No. 46. London: NICE, 2002.

Chapter 17

Resuscitation and emergencies

Ken Hines

All healthcare professionals who work in the community may occasionally be required to resuscitate a victim of a cardiopulmonary arrest. Sudden cardiac arrest, particularly from coronary heart disease, remains one of the most common causes of death. Many of these deaths occur outside hospital.

There is published evidence testifying to the effectiveness of healthcare professionals in providing early resuscitation and defibrillation, supported by the ambulance service in cases of ventricular fibrillation in the community. Properly equipped and trained primary care staff can do much to lower mortality in early acute myocardial infarction and in other medical emergencies presenting to general practice. Remember too that, on occasion, primary care staff may be called outside into the nearby street to assist at incidents ranging from falls in the street to serious road traffic collisions or even a shooting in a bank raid!

So how well prepared is your practice? Do you need to suggest improvements? Every practice should develop an emergencies procedure that takes into account the skills and abilities of all those working in the practice, from the senior partner to the most junior receptionist. There are many practices where, for some parts of the day at least, there are no clinical staff in the building and a receptionist would have to cope.

For many practices, the practice nurse is probably the best person to coordinate the responses to any incident and to maintain the necessary equipment and drugs. There should be a nominated person in every practice who leads on emergency care, with the responsibility for the purchase, maintenance and replacement of equipment and drugs.

A record of the training of all staff and an audit of performance and the completion of clinical/critical incident forms should also be under the remit of the nominated person. All clinical staff should have annual refresher training in basic life support as a minimum. Some staff may elect to have further training in advanced life support or other emergency training, depending on their interests and previous training and experience. Non-clinical staff in the practice should also be trained to basic life support standards, with a minimum of a refresher course every 2 years.

The reception staff may well have a vital role in the recognition and care of the emergency presenting first to the reception desk. Some receptionists could be encouraged to undertake a certified course in first aid as part of their personal career development.

In-house training based on role-play scenarios and asking 'What if?' can be great fun and will liven up any practice meeting. It will help to make reception staff feel part of the team.

EQUIPMENT

Ideally, to deal with cardiac arrest, every practice should acquire an automatic external defibrillator (AED). Indeed, it has been suggested that one should hang beside every fire extinguisher.

More and more AEDs are to be found in the community. Most supermarkets and department stores now have them and first-aid staff trained to use them. If, following a cardiac arrest in the surgery, somebody had to go down the road to borrow one from a supermarket there could be some red faces! Remember that it could be one of the staff who needs resuscitation rather than a member of the public. Ensure there is a supply of defibrillator pads.

Oxygen is now a must for every surgery, together with a delivery system capable of providing 15 litres a minute via an appropriate mask to give as near 100% oxygen as possible. The cylinder should be large enough to last for 15 minutes, until ambulance backup arrives.

Suction is also a must have for practices and should be portable and not rely on an electricity supply. Both battery- and hand-operated suction pumps are available. Suitable catheters are also required and, if battery operated, the batteries need to be kept fully charged.

A nebulizer is probably also an essential. This can be either battery, mains or oxygen powered. A supply of suitable nebulizer masks and chambers should be available for all ages.

AIRWAY MANAGEMENT

Expired air ventilation is the minimum standard expected and should be performed when necessary with a pocket mask incorporating a one-way valve to prevent secretions from the patient reaching the rescuer.

Where staff are proficient and experienced in using a bag and mask this is a useful addition to the resuscitation trolley. However, unless this equipment is used regularly, skills atrophy and more efficient ventilation will be obtained with the pocket mask. Time should not be wasted with inexperienced staff struggling to use a bag and mask. The bag and mask system may be used with two operators, one holding the mask in place and the other squeezing it. If a bag and mask are to be used then the oxygen supply should be attached.

Devices such as an oropharyngeal airway or 'guedel' are suitable for use outside hospital and a range of sizes should be kept for those appropriately trained in their use. Nasopharyngeal airways and the laryngeal mask may have a role in the management of the airway in unconscious patients. Special training is, however, required for their use, and normal general practice staff

> **BOX 17.1   Choking in babies and children**
>
> **Choking in a baby**
> - Only attempt to clear an obstruction if the baby is unable to breathe for himself. Never try to remove an obstruction by blindly putting your fingers in his mouth.
> - To relieve choking in a baby who cannot breathe for himself, lay the baby along your arm, head down. Using the heel of your hand give up to five smart blows between the shoulder blades. If this fails to clear the airway, turn the baby over and give up to five chest thrusts. Chest thrusts are performed in the same way as chest compressions, but should be sharper and at a slower rate, with each thrust trying to relieve the obstruction.
> - Check the mouth, carefully remove any obvious obstructions, and reassess breathing. If there is no breathing, attempt up to five rescue breaths. If these are unsuccessful, repeat the sequence of five back blows and five chest thrusts.
> - Do not perform abdominal thrusts on a baby, as these may damage internal organs.
>
> **Choking in children**
> - A child can be placed over your knee, head down, to deliver up to five back blows between the shoulder blades.
> - If this fails, turn the child over and give up to five chest thrusts. These are performed in the same way as chest compressions, but should be sharper and at a slower rate, with each thrust trying to relieve the obstruction.
> - If these also fail, and the child is not breathing, check the mouth and carefully remove any obvious obstruction. Then attempt up to five rescue breaths. If these are unsuccessful give five more back blows and then go on to give up to five abdominal thrusts with less force than for an adult. If this still fails, continue in cycles of five back blows, five chest thrusts, five rescue breaths, five back blows, five abdominal thrusts, five rescue breaths and so on.
>
> **A baby is a child under the age of 1 year, and a child is aged between 1 and 8 years of age.**
>
> *Resuscitation for the Citizen*, 6th edn. Resuscitation Council; 2000. Available at: http://www.resus.org

would not be expected to maintain proficiency in their use, unless trained in immediate pre-hospital emergency care and using the equipment regularly.

DRUGS

Epinephrine (adrenalin) has an established role in increasing the effectiveness of basic life support and is recommended in the current resuscitation guidelines. Atropine has an established role in the treatment of bradycardia, asystole and slow pulseless electrical activity (PEA). There is no established role for the use of alkalizing agents, buffers or calcium salts before hospital admission. Amiodarone is now recommended for refractory ventricular fibrillation or ventricular tachycardia.

All emergency drugs should be given via the intravenous route, preferably through a cannula placed in a large vein and flushed in with a bolus of intravenous fluid. To achieve this, a supply of intravenous cannulae, giving sets, tape and intravenous fluids, such as normal saline or Hartmann's solution, should be available on the resuscitation trolley.

Patient group directions for the administration of immunizations in general practice call for the provision of epinephrine to deal with the potential risk from anaphylaxis. Epinephrine is the first drug of choice here and can be administered by any trained clinician. It should be remembered, however, that patients may present with anaphylaxis caused by nut allergies or wasp stings and these are more common than reactions to vaccines. Ampoules of an antihistamine such as chlorpheniramine and hydrocortisone may subsequently also be used by a doctor in severe attacks.

Many practices use disease-specific packs to deal with acute medical events (Box 17.2), often packed in a 'Tupperware'-type box clearly labelled with the condition it is for and the earliest expiry date of any drugs included. Such packs are particularly useful for conditions such as acute left ventricular failure, prolonged seizures, meningitis, hypoglycaemia and acute myocardial infarction.

BOX 17.2   Emergency treatment packs

Diabetes
- Needles, syringes, intravenous cannulae and tape, pair of gloves
- Tube of Hypostop
- Two vials of glucagon and diluent
- Blood sugar testing kit and testing strips
- 50% glucose for intravenous administration is a last resort, but could be included if required

Angina/myocardial infarction
- Needles, syringes, intravenous cannulae and tape, pair of gloves
- GTN spray
- Aspirin 300 mg tabs
- Reminder that controlled drug analgesia is available from the locked cupboard

Acute heart failure
- Needles, syringes, intravenous cannulae and tape, pair of gloves
- Furosemide ampoules

Meningitis
- Needles, syringes, intravenous cannulae and tape, pair of gloves
- Dosage card for children
- Crystapen penicillin vials and diluent

Epilepsy
- Needles, syringes, intravenous cannulae and tape, pair of gloves
- Rectal diazepam
- Diazemol (intravenous diazepam)
- Lorazepam ampoules

Asthma
- Needles, syringes, intravenous cannulae and tape, pair of gloves
- Salbutamol inhaler
- Ipratropium bromide inhaler
- Steroid inhaler of choice
- Prednisolone 5 mg tabs
- Peak flow meter and mouth piece (adult and child)
- Salbutamol nebulizer solution
- Ipratropium nebulizer solution
- Hydrocortisone for intravenous injection
- Nebulizer and appropriate masks and chambers for adults and children

Infusion pack
- Two bottles of intravenous fluid, either saline or Hartmann's
- Selection of suitable cannulae
- Four giving sets
- Tape and bandages to secure giving line and cannulae
- Arm splint
- Scissors

PRACTICE PROTOCOLS

Practice meetings are the ideal time to rehearse how the practice would respond to an emergency in the building. Ask the question: 'What if?' What if a patient presents in the reception area with acute central chest pain? To whom should the staff in reception turn for help? Are they all confident in making 999 calls? Does the most junior and newest member of staff know where there is a cylinder of oxygen if sent to get it? Can non-clinical staff turn the cylinder on and use an appropriate flow rate?

An emergency can occur anywhere in the building, from the toilet to the car park – it is often not the treatment room or a consulting room, which can offer some privacy, but in full view of other patients in the premises. This means that all equipment and drugs required need to be easily portable and everyone must be able to identify what is required and take it to the required location.

Ask more questions. What if someone presents to the reception with an arterial bleed? Do the staff know the immediate first-aid reaction? Do they have any basic first-aid equipment in the reception area? What if a patient has a grand mal fit or even a simple faint in the waiting area? Are there facilities to screen the incident or somewhere to move other patients to?

True emergencies are rare in general practice. It is, however, prudent to be prepared. It is not satisfactory to rely on a 10-minute paramedic response to bail you out. Every practice has its fire procedures, and it is well worth the effort to have an emergency plan to deal with those rare clinical emergencies. One final consideration will be: what if the emergency involves the collapse of one of your own team? If an incident does occur, a critical incident report form should be completed. The event should be discussed at a practice meeting, actions and procedures reviewed, and documentation kept for use in appraisal and quality and outcome framework assessments.

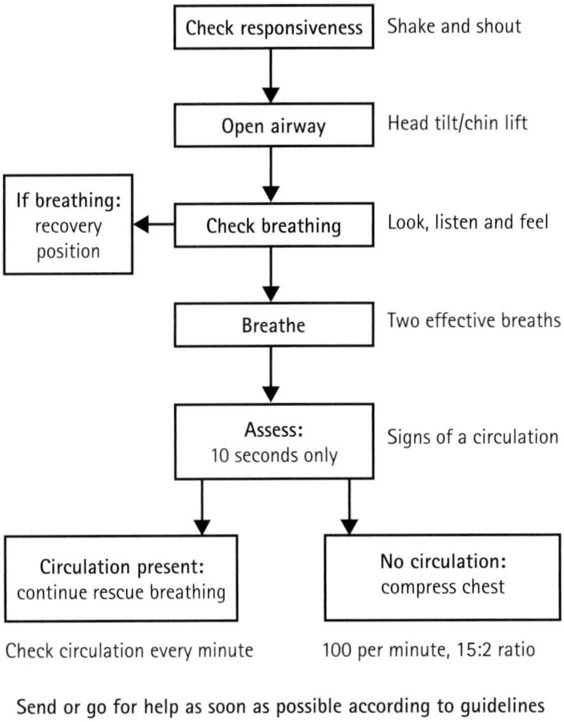

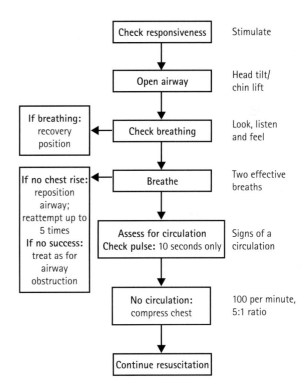

Send or go for help as soon as possible according to guidelines

Figure 17.1 Adult basic life support.

Send or go for help as soon as possible according to guidelines

Figure 17.2 Paediatric basic life support.

ESSENTIAL SKILLS

- Access the statutory BLS training via the local PCT
- Access the statutory anaphylaxis training via local PCT
- Read the patient group directions at the practice for all injections the nurse is likely to give
- Identify the location and condition of any resuscitation equipment held in the practice and familiarize yourself with it
- Check the location and content of the reception first-aid box
- Check the location and dates of any drugs held to deal with emergencies
- Check the location and battery condition of the defibrillator
- Ask questions about how the practice will deal with emergencies
- Find out if there is a chest pain procedure for reception staff

---

RESOURCES

Resuscitation Council UK: the Council website has a variety of algorithms for both basic and advanced life support for adults, children and neonates. These can be downloaded and kept in a suitable place for easy access if and when required. http://www.resus.org.uk

British Heart Foundation: the BHF website contains a lot of useful material for the practice nurse, some of which is useful to give to patients with coronary heart disease. http://www.bhf.org.uk

Heartstart Programme: this programme of community resuscitation training, coordinated by the BHF, is useful for non-clinical staff employed in a practice. Details of local schemes will be available from your PCT.

Chapter 18

Anaphylaxis and severe allergy

Sue Clarke

Severe allergic reactions, known as anaphylaxis, can be unpredictable. Families getting used to a diagnosis of anaphylaxis often feel overwhelmed with the enormity of trying to keep their child safe. Severe allergy management affects every part of the lives of those trying to deal with it, from the fundamentals of finding safe food to eat, to visiting family and friends, going on holiday, finding suitable childcare and schooling, to considering future career aspirations.

Practice nurses can play a vital part in helping families to manage this frightening condition, which is becoming more prevalent. Advisers to the Department of Health believe that about 1 million people are affected by acute severe allergy in the UK. Peanut allergy alone rose in incidence from 1:200 children in 1996 to 1:70 children in 2002.

WHAT IS ANAPHYLAXIS?

Anaphylaxis is a severe systemic allergic reaction. The whole body can be affected within minutes of exposure to the allergen, or it may be hours before effects are felt – although this is rare.[1]

There are many symptoms which can signify a reaction (Box 18.1). However for the reaction to be anaphylactic there would be one or both of two specific features:[2]

BOX 18.1   Symptoms that suggest an anaphylactic reaction

- Generalized flushing of the skin
- Nettle rash (hives or urticaria) anywhere on the body
- Sense of impending doom
- Swelling of the mouth and throat (angio-oedema)
- Difficulty in swallowing or speaking
- Alterations in heart rate
- Asthma
- Abdominal pain, nausea and vomiting
- Sudden feeling of weakness
- Collapse and unconsciousness

BOX 18.2   The allergens responsible for most anaphylactic reactions

- Peanut
- Tree nuts
- Milk and dairy products
- Egg
- Sesame
- Fish
- Shellfish
- Natural latex rubber
- Wasp and bee venom
- Penicillin

- difficulty breathing, including laryngeal oedema or asthma
- hypotension, including fainting or collapse and unconsciousness.

Severe allergic reactions can be caused by many things, but most reactions are caused by a few common allergens (Box 18.2).

Some mild reactions can be treated with quick-acting antihistamines. If the symptoms progress rapidly, then adrenalin (epinephrine) is the main treatment. It is highly effective and should be given by intramuscular injection without delay (Table 18.1).

Patients at risk of anaphylaxis should be prescribed adrenalin for self-administration. There are two autoinjectors available for this purpose:

- the Anapen
- the Epipen.

Both come in a paediatric dose of 0.15 mg adrenalin 1:1000, and an adult dose of 0.3 mg adrenalin 1:1000.

Anaphylaxis can also occur after routine immunizations and vaccinations, and some patients rush to the GP surgery when having an allergic reaction instead of calling an ambulance, so practice nurses need to know how to recognize the signs and give emergency treatment.

Emergency life-saving treatment can legally be given by the practice nurse if no doctor is on the premises, under Section 64 of the Medicines Act. However the nurse has a responsibility to ensure she has received adequate training in dealing with anaphylaxis. Regular anaphylaxis training is a prerequisite of patient group directions for the administration of immunizations and vaccinations in primary care.

AUTOINJECTOR TRAINING

If an autoinjector is prescribed, the patient and close family need to be trained in its use and also friends, school staff, babysitters, extended family

TABLE 18.1   Recommended adrenalin doses for the treatment of anaphylactic reaction

Age	Dose	Volume of adrenalin 1:1000 (1 mg/ml)
< 6 months	50 μg	0.05 ml
6 months–6 years	120 μg	0.12 ml
6–12 years	250 μg	0.25 ml
Adult and adolescent	500 μg	0.5 ml

Reproduced with permission from the Resuscitation Council UK[3]

etc. Most people are nervous about giving an injection, but are usually reassured once they have practised with a trainer pen (available from the manufacturer at a cost of about £6).

PATIENT ASSESSMENT

All patients whose symptoms suggest anaphylaxis should be referred to a specialist allergy clinic. Only by receiving an assessment can their risk be determined. Unfortunately there are few NHS allergy clinics in the UK, and families may have to wait months for an appointment. These families need support and information in the interim period. The Anaphylaxis Campaign provides this for families and health professionals through newsletters, fact sheets and a telephone helpline.

Adrenalin may need to be supplied before the specialist appointment. This can be a difficult decision. Once an autoinjector has been prescribed it is difficult to take away if the allergy is found to be mild. However, an autoinjector is likely to be needed if:

- previous reactions affected the airway or the circulation
- there is coexisting asthma
- the allergen suspected is peanut, nuts, seeds, shellfish or latex (these can have unpredictable effects).

ALLERGY EDUCATION

Families need to learn everything they can about the allergy in order to manage it successfully. Coexisting asthma increases the chances of a life-threatening reaction, so families should ensure asthma is well controlled.[4] Some allergy sufferers react to minute quantities of their allergen, including smelling the allergen or touching it, whilst others can tolerate close contact as long as they do not eat it.

FOOD SHOPPING

At first, food shopping can be difficult. As a starting point it is worth learning all the names that can apply to the allergen. For example, peanut can also be called earthnut, monkey nut, ground-nut or *Arachis*. Furthermore, a loophole in UK law called the '25% rule' allows some ingredients to remain legally undeclared on the wrapper. Many companies have realized how dangerous this is to those with allergies and now declare ingredients present in minute amounts. Other companies produce listings of products 'free from' certain ingredients which are available on request, although this means scanning pages of product information to find foods that can be eaten.

'May contain' labelling and cross-contamination are growing problems. Some products carry a genuine risk of cross-contamination (e.g. cornflakes made on the same production line as crunchy nut cornflakes). However, some manufacturers' labels carry a cross-contamination warning irrespective of the actual level of risk.

Some food manufacturers are leading the way in good practice. Kinnerton (http://www.Kinnerton.com) has divided its chocolate and confectionery factory so that certain products can be guaranteed nut free.

DOMESTIC CROSS-CONTAMINATION

Cross-contamination can occur in the home too. Some families deal with this risk by banning the allergen from the home, but this is not always possible, particularly when dealing with multiple food allergies. Families can reduce the risk by preparing allergenic food in a separate area of the kitchen and by scrupulous washing-up procedures. Visiting other families can present further risks. For example, nuts and seeds from indoor pet foods or outdoor bird feeders can be an unforeseen hazard. Similarly, many children enjoy peanut butter and jam sandwiches, so watch out for contaminated jars of jam.

EATING OUT

Thai, Indonesian and Indian foods are not suitable for nut allergy sufferers. Simple foods like steak, and chicken and chips with salad are often the safest choice. Clear communication is essential, and it is safer to speak to the chef directly rather than rely on a waiter to pass on information.

HOLIDAYS

Holidays should be planned with precision, especially if travelling abroad. Some airlines will supply special dietary meals, but these can be unreliable. It is safer to pack a personal food supply for the journey. If the allergy sufferer reacts to the smell of nuts it is worth asking for a 'nut-free' flight. With the current high levels of airline security, you should also check in advance that autoinjectors are allowed in hand baggage.

Self-catering accommodation is available in most countries, allowing families to combine simple local produce with foods they have brought from home. When shopping on holiday, a dictionary and translation cards are useful to explain the allergy. If travelling with a tour operator, a representative who speaks the local language could check out the local bakeries.

AGE-SPECIFIC ISSUES

Specific everyday problems arise at different stages of childhood, and listening to the experiences of other families speeds the process of finding solutions. The Anaphylaxis Campaign has a network of regional contacts throughout the UK, who can link families up to exchange ideas.

Babies and toddlers

Babies and toddlers have no sense of danger and carers must think for them to ensure their safety.

If toys are shared, for example at a playgroup, they can become contaminated with food, and at this age everything is liable to be put into the mouth. If allergic reactions occur, the child may need toys solely for his or her own use, to avoid further reactions.

Babies with allergies are likely to be breast-fed, or fed on an extensively hydrolysed formula. Care should be taken, especially in nurseries, to ensure they are always given the correct milk. Most manufactured baby foods in the UK are well labelled. However, when the child moves on to family meals, all the previously discussed hazards of shopping for safe food apply.

Pre-schoolers

Pre-schoolers are taught not to touch a hot stove; similarly, they can be taught that food must be checked by a trusted adult before eating. They can start to recognize foods that should be avoided, and spot simple words such as 'nut', 'milk' and 'egg'.

School-age children

As children get older they want to go to parties on their own. This can be difficult for parents, but if they have been teaching their child how to manage the allergy since pre-school, they can be confident their child will not take risks.

An adult who is competent to manage the allergy must be present at the party. For children allergic to just nuts or peanuts the party-giver may be prepared to ensure all the food is nut free, but children with multiple food allergies will need to take their own food along.

Children develop busy lives outside the home, attending groups and activities. Parents are expected to leave their children and collect them later. The adults in charge must understand about allergy, what causes the reaction, how they can prevent it, how to administer emergency treatment and how to summon help.

Peer pressure and bullying could be issues for school-age children. There is no easy answer to bullying, but encouraging children to include their friends in their allergy management can help.

The teenage years

As teenagers move toward independence, they increasingly socialize without their parents. They should be able to teach their friends what foods they can safely eat, how to use the autoinjector and what to do in an emergency.

Organized group outings, such as school trips, should not automatically be ruled out. With careful planning many teenagers with allergies can join in, especially if they can organize and cook their own food.

Teenagers must be aware that kissing someone who has been eating foods that they are allergic to can be dangerous. Explaining this to a new boyfriend or girlfriend can be embarrassing, but is vitally important. They must also understand that alcohol affects judgement and can speed up an allergic reaction. The implications of getting drunk are more serious than a sore head next day.

CAREER PLANNING

Some careers are not open to allergic young people – for example, joining the armed forces, or becoming a commercial airline pilot or a chef. However, allergic youngsters have usually developed special skills, such as self-reliance, confidence, assertiveness and empathy, which can be useful in many careers.

CONCLUSION

Anaphylaxis is a frightening condition, but it is manageable. Families may initially need a great deal of help, support and practical advice. They should be encouraged to have regular training updates with autoinjector trainer pens, and to practise their emergency procedure every few months.

The Anaphylaxis Campaign can update families on new developments in allergy management with its publications, helpline and website.

Many parents react by taking control of their child's environment. The allergen is removed from the house, all foods are checked before eating and the emergency medication looked after by the parents. This is a natural reaction to a stressful situation, but not always in the best interests of the child. Even young children can take some responsibility for their allergy. Learning to handle an allergy under supervision can alleviate fear and empower them.

ESSENTIAL SKILLS

- Recognize the signs and symptoms of anaphylaxis
- Know how to treat and get further help
- Undertake annual anaphylaxis training
- Ensure there is an up-to-date anaphylaxis kit available
- Know how to demonstrate autoinjector use
- Know where to get further information about anaphylaxis
- Work within agreed patient group directions and PCT policies for anaphylaxis

---

REFERENCES

1. Fisher M McD. Clinical observations on the pathophysiology and treatment of anaphylactic cardiovascular collapse. Anaesth Intens Care 1998; 14: 17–21.

2. Ewan P. ABC of Allergies: anaphylaxis. BMJ 1998; 316: 1442–1445.

3. Resuscitation Council UK. The Emergency Medical Treatment of an Anaphylactic Reaction for First Medical

Responders and for Community Nurses. A Project Team Report (revised January 2002). Available at: http://www.resus.org.uk/pages/ reaction.htm

4. Sampson HA, Mendelson L, Rosen JP. Fatal and near fatal reactions to food in children and adolescents. N Engl J Med 1992; 327: 380–384.

USEFUL WEBSITES

Anaphylaxis Campaign: Tel. 01252 542029; http://www.anaphylaxis.org.uk

Allergy in Schools: Tel. 01252 542029; http://www.allergyinschools.org.uk

Allergy UK: Tel. 01322 619864; http://www.allergyuk.org.uk

Latex Allergy Support Group: Tel. 07071 225838 (7–10 p.m.); http://www.lasg.co.uk

Epipen: provides information for families about using an Epipen. Health professionals can order a patient training kit. http://www.epipen.co.uk

Section 2

Disease management

SECTION CONTENTS

Diabetes

Gwen Hall

There are currently 1.3 million people diagnosed with diabetes, with this number set to double in 10 years. Diabetes UK, the national charity involving people with diabetes, is concerned about 'the missing millions' of undiagnosed sufferers.

There is a wealth of evidence that systematic and effective care limits the potentially devastating effects of diabetes. However, to date diabetes is still the largest cause of kidney failure, the leading cause of blindness in adults of working age and one of the biggest causes of lower-limb amputation.

About 75% of people with type 2 diabetes will die of cardiovascular disease.[1] Yet we know that type 2 diabetes is largely preventable;[2] healthy diet, increasing activity and maintaining an ideal body weight all play their part; but the King's Fund report saw no grounds for optimism that the necessary far-reaching changes in the population's lifestyle will be achieved.

WHAT IS DIABETES?

There are two main types of diabetes: type 1 (which used to be referred to as insulin-dependent diabetes or juvenile-onset diabetes) and type 2 (previously called non-insulin-dependent diabetes or maturity-onset diabetes). Between 75% and 80% of people with diabetes will have type 2 and most will be in the older age brackets. However, type 2 diabetes is on the increase in younger people, especially the obese, and we do see type 1 developing in older people. Just because someone with type 2 diabetes may be treated with insulin does not make them a type 1 diabetes patient (Box 19.1).

Type 1 diabetes

In type 1 diabetes an autoimmune process is frequently implicated in the destruction of the beta cells in the pancreas. This results in a rapidly diminishing output of insulin and a consequent elevation of blood sugar, leading to symptoms and eventual ketoacidosis if not detected and treated swiftly. These patients invariably require referral to the specialist diabetes team and will not be dealt with here.

Type 2 diabetes

Type 2 diabetes has a more insidious onset. There is gradual deterioration in the body's response to the available insulin due to insulin resistance, and secondary failure of the beta cells may develop

(Figure 19.1). These people are frequently managed in primary care and the rest of this chapter focuses on their care.

THE SYMPTOMS OF DIABETES

The symptoms of each type reflect the condition (Box 19.2). A high level of suspicion of diabetes should be maintained at all times in people displaying any of these symptoms.[3]

WHOM SHOULD WE SCREEN?

Type 2 diabetes is largely responsible for the rising incidence of diabetes. Increasing sedentary lifestyles at all ages, rising levels of obesity and the ability to live longer all contribute. It is not necessary to screen the whole population for diabetes but, again, it is wise to adopt a high level of suspicion in the groups listed in Box 19.3 and screen them, normally with a laboratory blood or urine test.[4] Be aware that urine tests in elderly people may not be effective because of their high renal threshold.

BOX 19.1 Differentiating features of diabetes	
Type 1	Type 2
Rapid onset	Slow onset
Age < 30 years at diagnosis (but can be older)	Age > 30 years at diagnosis (but can be younger)
History of unplanned weight loss	Often overweight/obese
Beta cell destruction	Beta cell deterioration/insulin resistance
Positive family history in 10% of cases	Positive family history in 30% of cases
50% concordance in identical twins	100% concordance in identical twins
Insulin essential	Healthy eating and keeping up activity levels are the keys to control, with tablets and/or insulin to control blood glucose levels. Strongly linked to heart disease

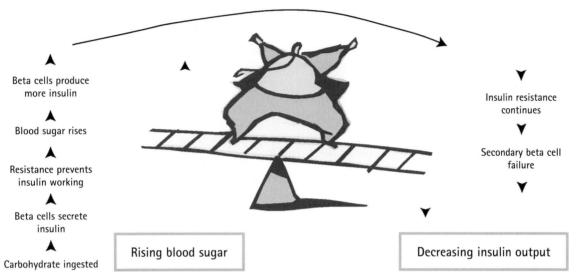

Beta cells produce
more insulin

Blood sugar rises

Resistance prevents
insulin working

Beta cells secrete
insulin

Carbohydrate ingested

Insulin resistance
continues

Secondary beta cell
failure

Rising blood sugar

Decreasing insulin output

Figure 19.1   Insulin resistance.

DIAGNOSIS

If a patient is symptomatic and has a blood sugar reading in the diabetic range a diagnosis can be confirmed (Box 19.4). For those without symptoms a further check, on a subsequent day, should be performed to confirm the diagnosis.

There are local variations in performing tests for diabetes. Glucose levels may be tested at random, with the length of time since the last meal being recorded. Alternatively, blood glucose is tested after the patient has fasted overnight (10–16 hours), during which time only water should be drunk.

If the random test or test following fasting does not prove diagnostic, then the 2-hour oral glucose tolerance test (OGTT) should be carried out. For this test the patient must eat a normal diet containing carbohydrates for at least 3 days and then fast overnight.If the blood test following fasting does not confirm the diagnosis, then a 75 g glucose load (seek advice on this from your local laboratory) is taken by the patient and the blood test repeated after 2 hours. The patient should be advised that smoking is not permitted during the test period and you should record it if this is not adhered to.

Any child in whom a diagnosis is suspected should be referred urgently by telephone to a hospital paediatric department, where the diagnosis can be confirmed.

BOX 19.2 Symptoms suggestive of diabetes		
Type 1	**Type 2**	**Both**
• Rapid onset	• Insidious onset	• Thirst
• Often marked weight loss	• May have weight loss	• Polyuria
• Hunger and/or abdominal pain	• Pins and needles/numbness in extremities	• Vaginal thrush
		• Changes to vision
		• Lethargy/irritation
		• Recurrent infections

BOX 19.3 Whom should we screen?

Those presenting with the following symptoms:
- Thirst, polyuria and weight loss
- Nocturia, incontinence
- Recurrent infections, leg ulcers, thrush
- Neuropathic symptoms, e.g. pain, numbness and paraesthesia
- Visual changes such as blurring of vision
- Lassitude and general malaise
- Confusion – especially in the elderly

Those already attending with:
- Hypertension
- Ischaemic heart disease
- Peripheral vascular disease
- Cerebrovascular disease

All pregnant women

BOX 19.4 Diagnostic criteria

Diabetes
- Fasting glucose > 7 mmol/l *or*
- Non-fasting glucose > 11 mmol/l

Impaired glucose tolerance (IGT)
- Fasting glucose > 6.4 mmol/l *and*
- 2 hours after glucose load > 7.8 mmol/l but < 11.1 mmol/l

Impaired fasting glucose (IFG)
- Fasting glucose > 6.1 mmol/l but < 7 mmol/l

CURRENT TREATMENT

First and foremost this is a healthy lifestyle.

Healthy eating plan

The word 'diet' may strike dread into many of us! Nurses in primary care should recognize the contribution of a dietitian to the team and be prepared to tailor advice to individuals and their treatment. If you do not have a dietitian visiting the practice where you work, find out if it is possible to sit in on a local session or seek up-to-date training. Establish what your local referral policy regarding dietitians involves.

ACTIVITY

Activity is as important as a good diet. Walking briskly for 30 minutes five times a week is suggested as the minimum level to obtain health benefits. Obviously this needs tailoring to the

individual – an overweight fit person is probably in a better state of health than an unfit thin one.[5]

Many newly diagnosed people with type 2 diabetes are obese. The tendency is towards central obesity – apple shaped rather than pear shaped – which is an indicator of risk not only of type 2 diabetes but also of cardiovascular disease and stroke.

MEDICATION

The DARTS study stressed that about half of patients with diabetes do not take all their medication as we might think they do. Many are on therapy for blood pressure, lipids and diabetes (Table 19.1).[6] This polypharmacy does not engender compliance, and a simple question to patients is 'Tell me what medication you're currently taking and when'. It is an eye opener!

Although it is not within the scope of this chapter, practice nurses should make themselves aware of the broad range of medication someone with diabetes may be taking.

Hypos – unwanted side-effect of medication

The American Diabetes Control & Complications Trial (DCCT)[7] demonstrated that strict control of blood glucose in type 1 patients lessens the risks associated with diabetes complications. Hypos in

TABLE 19.1   Drug treatments for diabetes

Drug type	Name	Mode of action	Comments
Sulphonylureas	Glibenclamide Tolbutamide Gliclazide	Increases beta cell insulin secretion	Longer acting agents, such as Glibenclamide, contraindicated in the elderly
Biguanides	Metformin	Decreases glucose output from liver and increases cellular response to insulin	First drug of choice in the overweight but may cause transient gastric disturbances and should be started at a low dose
α-Glucosidase inhibitors	Acarbose	Reduces postprandial glucose peak by inhibiting gastrointestinal carbohydrate digestion	May cause initial gastric disturbances, and care must be used in treating hypos if used in conjunction with sulphonylureas
Thiazolidine diones	Rosiglitazone Pioglitazone	Improves insulin sensitivity	Regular liver function monitoring required
Postprandial glucose regulators	Repaglinide Nateglinide	Reduces blood glucose rise after meals through short, rapid action	Fast-acting tablet taken before meals to regulate blood glucose. May be added to Metformin

those patients have been described as 'unavoidable', yet, along with the fear of possible complications, they are the most feared aspect of diabetes to those who have to live with the disease.[6–8] People with type 2 diabetes can be at risk too if they are treated with sulphonylureas (Glibenclamide and Chlorpropamide in particular, although the latter is rarely used nowadays) and may suffer from protracted hypos due to the lengthy duration of action of the medication.[9] Make sure these patients are given information on prevention.

TREATMENT TARGETS

Diabetes UK suggests good, borderline and poor targets for diabetes management (Table 19.2). It should be borne in mind that these targets are not achievable and not appropriate for all. People with diabetes need to be involved in deciding what changes they wish to make to help them achieve their targets. Health professionals need to consider the individual and tailor their care to suit.

MANAGEMENT

The nurse new to diabetes management should beware of taking on too much. Diabetes is a highly complex condition and support from colleagues will be invaluable until specific training has been undertaken.

Care should be involved in the formation of an acceptable protocol or pathway. Diabetes reviews can generally be categorized into:

- new patient
- routine review
- annual review.

Who does what within a protocol may vary, but involvement of the patient in his or her own care is paramount. After all it is the patient who provides the care, while the nurse's role is to give them the tools to do the job.

Management plans

For detailed management plans that can be adapted to local need, get acquainted with the

TABLE 19.2   Recommendations for the management of diabetes in primary care

	Targets for metabolic control and the control of cardiovascular risk factors in people with diabetes		
	Good[a]	Borderline	Poor
Plasma glucose (mmol/l): fasting	4.4–6.1	6.2–7.8	> 7.8
Plasma glucose (mmol/l): postprandial	4.4–8.0	8.1–10.0	> 10.0
HbA_{1c}[a] (%)	< 6.5	6.5–7.5	> 7.5
Urine glucose (%)	0	0–0.5	> 0.5
Total cholesterol (mmol/l)	< 5.2	5.2–6.5	> 6.5
HDL cholesterol (mmol/l)	> 1.1	0.9–1.1	< 0.9
Fasting triglycerides (mmol/l)	< 1.7	1.7–2.2	> 2.2
Body mass index (kg/m^2): males	20–25	26–27	> 27
Body mass index (kg/m^2): females	19–24	25–26	> 26
Blood pressure (mmHg)	< 140/80[b, c]	140/80–160/95	> 160/95
Smoking	Non-smoker	Pipe smoker	Cigarettes

[a]Reference ranges for HbA_{1c} vary greatly depending on the assay method used – some laboratories still measure total HbA_1. You should check the reference range in the laboratory that you use. The values given in the table assume that normal HbA_{1c} is < 6.1%.
[b]Stricter targets are necessary in younger people and in people with early nephropathy who have a good life expectancy.
[c]Following the results of the UKPDS, Diabetes UK now recommends that blood pressure above 140/80 should be treated.

Diabetes UK document *Recommendations for the Management of Diabetes in Primary Care* (available at: http://www. diabetes.org.uk).

Patients should also be encouraged to be actively involved in their own management, for example by using patient-held records (Box 19.5).

NATIONAL SERVICE FRAMEWORK

The National Service Framework (NSF) for Diabetes: Standards and Delivery Strategy, published in 2001 and 2002, set out the objectives for diabetes management until 2013. A visit to the NSF website (http://www.doh.gov.uk/nsf/diabetes)

BOX 19.5   Information included in a personal diabetes record

- An agreed care plan, including education and the personal goals of the person with diabetes
- How their diabetes is to be managed until their next review; this fosters greater understanding and ownership of the goals of diabetes care
- Health, social care and education needs, how they will be met and who will be responsible
- The named contact

is well worthwhile, as it contains more than the printed articles themselves.

ESSENTIAL SKILLS

- Understand the difference between type 1 and type 2 diabetes
- Be confident with strategies to prevent diabetes and its complications, especially coronary heart disease
- Recognize factors enabling patients to take effective medication
- Know where to obtain current advice on diabetes management and put it into practice through your professional learning plan
- Be able to participate in a planned programme of care involving people with diabetes

REFERENCES

1. Kings Fund. Counting the Cost. The Real Impact of Non Insulin Dependent Diabetes. London: Kings Fund/Diabetes UK (formerly British Diabetic Association), 1996.
2. Department of Health. 2002 National Service Framework for Diabetes. Research. Epidemiology and Primary Prevention. Available at: http://www.dh.gov.uk
3. Diabetes UK. Recommendations for the Management of Diabetes in Primary Care. London: Diabetes UK, 2000. Available at: http://www.diabetes.org.uk
4. Meakin J. Active Benefits. Diabetes Update Spring Fact Sheet 16. London: BDA (now Diabetes UK), 2000.
5. Donnan PT, MacDonald TM, Morris AD. Adherence to prescribed oral hypoglycaemic medication in a population of patients with type 2 diabetes: a retrospective cohort study. Diabetic Med 2002; 19: 279–284.
6. Working Party Report. Diabetes & Cognitive Function: The Evidence So Far. London: BDA (now Diabetes UK), 1996.
7. DCCT Research Group. The effect of intensive treatment of diabetes on the development and progression of long-term complications in insulin-dependent diabetes mellitus. N Engl J Med 1993; 329: 977–986.
8. Frier BM. Morbidity of hypoglycaemia. Diabetes Rev Intl 1994; 3(2).
9. Sinclair AJ, Turnbull CJ, Croxson SCM. Document of care for older people with diabetes. Postgrad Med J 1996; 72: 334–338.

Chapter 20

Diabetes: hypo- and hyperglycaemic attacks

Gwen Hall

To understand hypo- and hyperglycaemic states we need a short recap on diabetes. When glucose is ingested it is absorbed into the bloodstream and the blood glucose level rises. In a person who does not have diabetes this stimulates the beta cells (situated in the pancreas) to produce insulin. This in turn stimulates cells to take in this glucose for later use. The muscles and liver also store glucose as glycogen – a ready source of energy in times of need. These actions take the glucose out of the blood and the glucose level drops to normal. Should the level of glucose in the blood fall, due to lack of food or increased activity perhaps, the alpha cells (also in the pancreas) release glucagon, liberating glucose from the liver, and the balance is again returned to normal (Figure 20.1).

For the purposes of this chapter we will split diabetes into two distinct groups: type 1, where the body fails to produce insulin; and type 2, where the body may still produce insulin but insulin resistance prevents it working. In type 1 diabetes, treatment always includes insulin along with healthy eating and maintenance of activity. In type 2 diabetes, treatment consists of healthy eating to attempt to achieve an ideal body weight, continuing activity, introduction of one or more tablets and, in worsening cases, initiation of insulin.

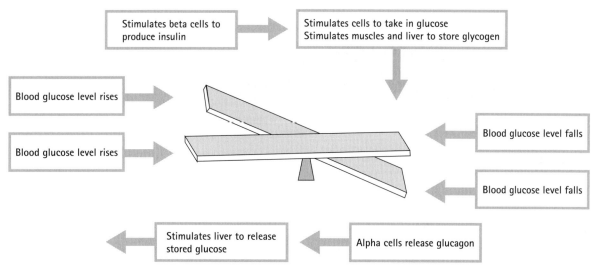

Figure 20.1   Release of insulin and glucagon from the alpha and beta cells.

HYPERGLYCAEMIA – HIGH BLOOD GLUCOSE

It is generally accepted that hyperglycaemia occurs when the level of glucose in the blood rises above 10 mmol/l.[1] This can be checked on a blood glucose meter that has been subject to quality assurance control to ensure it is reading correctly. Ask a trained colleague or specialist nurse if you are unsure about this.

Hyperglycaemia is frequently found in primary care in people with type 2 diabetes. It is difficult to achieve the tight control we advocate – blood glucose levels of 4–8 mmol/l before meals or an HbA_{1c} (long-term blood glucose test representing 3 months' control) of 7% or less.

Many patients will have had high glucose levels in their blood for a protracted period before diagnosis – years before may not be unusual. There is generally no emergency here – treatment and support to reduce glucose levels gradually is required, plus continuing support to prevent the progressive nature of the condition, allowing glucose levels to rise again untreated. Anyone with continuing elevated blood glucose levels needs review by their GP or diabetes trained nurse, and the higher the level

the quicker the review is needed. Blood glucose levels above the mid-teens, or an elevated HbA_{1c}, should be investigated and treated as a matter of urgency.

An elevated blood glucose level becomes an emergency in new or uncontrolled type 1 diabetes, where it can be the harbinger of diabetic ketoacidosis (Box 20.1). An absence of insulin causes very high blood glucose levels, resulting in fat and protein metabolism and the formation of ketone bodies, which can be detected in the urine (with Ketostix) or on the breath (if you can smell pear drops). The new practice nurse is unlikely to see this state, as it presents as a diabetic emergency and urgent hospital admission is essential.

BOX 20.1   Symptoms of diabetic ketoacidosis

- Nausea, vomiting
- Confusion, drowsiness, coma
- Abdominal pain
- Air hunger
- Weight loss
- Muscle cramps

Causes

High blood glucose levels will be found at diagnosis, but poor control, illness, inadequate medication and stress may cause hyperglycaemia (Box 20.2).

Symptoms

In mild hyperglycaemia the symptoms are generally similar to those often seen at diagnosis (Box 20.3). If it is progressing to diabetic keto-acidosis the symptoms worsen.

What to do

In mild to moderate hyperglycaemia, review of medication, diet and activity levels with a trained health professional is paramount. Some questions may uncover the cause:

- Is the healthy eating plan being adhered to?
- Could food with a hidden sugar content be responsible?
- Have activity levels decreased recently?
- Is there any infection present?
- Is the patient taking their medication as prescribed?

If there is no obvious cause, a medication review is required urgently. If you have not yet had the training to enable you to handle this subject confidently, refer to a senior nurse or GP.

Severe hyperglycaemia always requires urgent referral, whether type 1 or type 2.

HYPOGLYCAEMIA – LOW BLOOD GLUCOSE

Hypoglycaemia is commonly agreed to exist when blood glucose levels drop below 3 mmol/l. Remember, however, that 'hypo' symptoms dev-

---

> **BOX 20.2   Causes of hyperglycaemia**
>
> - Undiagnosed diabetes
> - Illness
> - Other medications that affect blood glucose (thiazide diuretics, steroids)
> - Increased sugar intake, decreased activity
> - Missed medication, especially insulin
> - Stress

> **BOX 20.3   Symptoms of hyperglycaemia**
>
> - Frequency of urine or passing large amounts (polyuria)
> - Lethargy
> - Possible changes to vision
> - Thirst
> - Irritability

elop at higher levels in response to a sudden drop in glucose levels, and the person who complains of symptoms at 10 mmol/l should not have these worries dismissed if their previous levels were up at 18 or 20 mmol/l.[1]

Hypos in those with type 1 diabetes have been described as 'unavoidable'.[2] And yet, along with fear of possible complications, they are the most feared aspect of diabetes to those who have to live with the disease.[3]

It is not only those with type 1 diabetes who are at risk. Patients treated with sulphonylureas (Glibenclamide and Chlorpropamide in particular, although the latter is rarely used nowadays) may suffer from protracted hypos due to the lengthy duration of action of the medication.[4] Other sulphonylureas (Gliclazide, Glimepiride) have a shorter action and are less implicated, but still they can cause hypos.

The brain relies on glucose to function. In diabetes treated with insulin or sulphonylureas, this essential supply can be artificially reduced – after all, the treatment is given to lower the blood glucose. It is this restriction of glucose to the brain that causes many of the symptoms of hypoglycaemia.

Causes

There are a number of factors that can lead to a hypo (Box 20.4). A detailed history is required to assist in investigating the cause of the hypo in order to prevent further attacks.

Symptoms

We rely on patients to detect hypos, but not everyone gets symptoms or warning signs – for example, those with autonomic neuropathy. The longer someone has diabetes the more likely they are to lose these valuable signs. Also, if someone has the perfect control we are all advocating, they may be less likely to detect hypos since their normal levels are so near to 4 mmol/l and their body may not respond to such a small drop in glucose level. The more hypos a person with diabetes has, the more they are likely to continue to have, unless the source can be identified and tackled.

Symptoms can be broken down into two main categories (Box 20.5) but what the patient, or more often their carers, will report is feeling and behaving quite differently from usual. A hypoglycaemic attack may be mistaken for drunkenness, and it is advisable for the person with diabetes to carry identification at all times to prevent misunderstanding about this (albeit unusual) occurrence.

BOX 20.4   Causes of hypoglycaemia

- Delayed or too little food
- Too much medication (either insulin or sulphonylureas)
- Reducing doses of drugs (e.g. steroids) that enhance oral hypoglycaemic agents
- Hot weather, which can speed up the action of insulin
- Unexpected increase in activity (strenuous activity can have an effect on blood glucose well into the next day)
- Overdose of medication (inadvertent or intentional)
- A change to a new injection site in someone who has developed an injection pad (lipohypertrophy) at one site due to overuse. Insulin will be better absorbed from a fresh site
- 'Hypos' can be exacerbated by alcohol

BOX 20.5   Symptoms of hypoglycaemia*

Autonomic or neurogenic – nervous system stimulation
- Sweating
- Hunger
- Trembling/shakiness
- Anxiety
- Palpitations/tachycardia

Neuroglycopenic – altered brain function
- Confusion
- Unusual behaviour
- Poor concentration
- Drowsiness
- Poor coordination
- Visual disturbance
- Tingling around the mouth

Others
- Weakness
- Nausea
- Dry mouth
- Headache

*Individual reactions will differ in onset and severity. Older patients may present with abnormal behaviour or impaired consciousness, which may be protracted if on long-acting sulphonylureas. Blood glucose control should be assessed before jumping to conclusions regarding their behaviour.

Although probably the province of the experienced nurse in diabetes, it is as well to know about the Somogyi effect. This is insulin-induced hypoglycaemia in the night which causes a 'rebound' hyperglycaemia in the morning. This should always be excluded before altering treatment based purely on early morning blood glucose readings.[5]

What to do

- Educate the patient to recognize and avoid the problem.
- Have something sugary to hand.
- If possible, check that the patient's glucose level is low, but do not delay treatment. It is always best to treat a possible hypo and ask questions later.

MILD HYPOGLYCAEMIA

In mild hypoglycaemia the person themselves or their carer will detect the problem, and should understand not only how to recognize it but also how to treat it appropriately. Do not encourage patients experiencing a hypo to make a cup of sugary tea (as some do), as the last thing you want is a person with shaky hands, not in full control of their faculties, boiling a kettle. Lucozade, cola, honey or any sugary drink (not reduced calorie) will do. This should be backed up with some longer acting carbohydrate; a sandwich or a meal if it is due, perhaps.

MODERATE HYPOGLYCAEMIA

If the patient is groggy but still awake Hypostop gel (on prescription) can be squeezed into the mouth, where it is absorbed from the buccal membranes. Honey can have the same effect but not so readily. Again this should be followed up with more solid food when the patient has recovered.

SEVERE HYPOGLYCAEMIA

The new practice nurse is unlikely to see this but patients and their carers need to be educated in its recognition and treatment. The patient is unconscious or unrousable. Medical attention should be sought and an ambulance called. In type 1 diabetes an injection of glucagon, either by the trained carer or a health professional, should be given. If this has the desired effect, and if the carer is competent, the patient may be managed at home on the advice of a doctor.

In type 2 diabetes, due to the prolonged action of sulphonylureas, if they are being taken, hospital admission is advisable.

ESSENTIAL SKILLS

- Be able to recognize the symptoms of hyperglycaemia and hypoglycaemia, and when and to whom to refer
- Be able to safely use a blood glucose meter with due regard to checking its reliability (quality assurance) and those used in patients' home monitoring
- Be able to advise patients/carers on recognition and treatment of hyperglycaemia
- Be able to advise patients/carers on recognition and treatment of hypoglycaemia
- Know where to get further advice

REFERENCES

1. MacKinnon M. Providing Diabetes Care in General Practice. London: Class, 2001.
2. Working Party Report. Diabetes & Cognitive Function: The Evidence So Far. London: BDA, 1996.
3. Frier BM. Morbidity of hypoglycaemia. Diabetes Rev Int 1994; 3(2).
4. Sinclair AJ, Turnbull CJ, Croxson SCM. Document of care for older people with diabetes. Postgrad Med J 1996; 72: 334–338.
5. Campbell I, Lebovitz H. Diabetes Mellitus: Fast Facts. Oxford: Health Press, 1996.

USEFUL WEBSITES

Diabetes UK has a number of useful publications available ('Balance for Beginners'; 'Hypoglycaemia'; 'Understanding Diabetes') and produces recommendations for the management of diabetes in primary care: Tel. 020 7424 1000; Fax: 020 7424 1001; http://www.diabetes.org.uk

Novo Nordisk Ltd has produced 'Help with Hypos' (free to health professionals): Customer Care Centre Tel. 0845 600 5055; http://www.novonordisk.co.uk

Aventis has produced 'What is a Hypo?' (free to health professionals): Tel. 01732 584000; http://www.aventis.co.uk

Chapter 21

Asthma care

Rachel Booker

Asthma is a chronic inflammatory condition of the airways, associated with variable airflow obstruction and an increase in response to a variety of stimuli. Obstruction is often reversible, either spontaneously or with treatment.[1]

It affects 5 million people in the UK and is the most common chronic disease of childhood.[2] A GP with a list of 2,500 patients can expect 125 of these to have asthma.

PATHOLOGY

There are three main aspects of airway inflammation:

- *Mucosal oedema* – swelling of the airway lining reduces airway calibre, and inflammatory cells (mast cells, basophils, neutrophils, macrophages and eosinophils) manufacture chemical mediators that perpetuate inflammation, cause bronchial hyperreactivity (BHR) and destroy airway epithelium.
- *Bronchospasm* – narrowing of the bronchi by muscle contraction in response to stimuli gives rise to symptoms of chest tightness and wheeze. The involuntary muscle surrounding the airway is abnormally 'twitchy', which is known as BHR.
- *Increased mucus* – sputum in asthma is often tacky and stained yellow or green by the inflammatory cells it contains. It is difficult to

clear, and in fatal asthma mucus plugs occlude some airways completely.

PRESENTATION

Asthma can present at any age but does so most commonly in childhood. Symptoms of cough, wheeze, chest tightness and shortness of breath on exertion can occur alone or in combination. Typically these symptoms are variable and intermittent, but nocturnal disturbance with cough and wheeze and symptoms that are worse on exertion or following viral upper respiratory tract infections (URTIs) are highly suggestive of asthma.

TRIGGERS

The most common trigger is URTI (Box 21.1). Colds 'go to the chest' and take several weeks to resolve. Exercise also triggers symptoms and many untreated asthmatics, consciously or unconsciously, avoid vigorous exercise.

Asthma that presents in childhood is often triggered by allergy to pollen, house dust mite or dander from animals such as cats and dogs or birds. Sufferers often have other allergic (atopic) conditions, such as eczema, hay fever or chronic rhinitis, and many have a positive family history of asthma. Occupational asthma typically improves during periods away from work, and suspected cases need specialist referral.

DIAGNOSIS

Diagnosis should be confirmed objectively before long-term treatment is started.[3]

Spirometry and peak expiratory flow

Spirometry or peak expiratory flow (PEF) is the preferred method. Spirometry requires special training but PEF is easy to perform. Predicted PEF levels are determined by height, age and sex in adults and height in children. In adults, levels up to 100 l/min above or below predicted can be considered normal in asymptomatic subjects.

Reversibility testing

Asthma can be confirmed by reversing airflow obstruction with a dose of bronchodilator or, in adults, with a course of oral steroids (Box 21.2). A positive result is a rise in PEF of 20% and at least 60 l/min from baseline (Box 21.3).[3]

Exercise testing

Most asthmatics experience bronchospasm following vigorous exercise, and this forms the

---

BOX 21.1   Asthma triggers

Allergens
- House dust mite
- Cat dander
- Other furry or feathered animals
- Foods (rare)
- Occupational 'sensitizers' (e.g. flour (bakers), isocyanates (plastics, foam rubber, paints), platinum salts (refinery workers), resins (glues, solders), enzymes (detergent manufacturing), laboratory animals)

Others
- Viral URTI
- Exercise
- Cold air
- Laughing, hyperventilating
- Drugs (beta blockers, non-steroidal anti-inflammatory drugs (NSAIDs), aspirin)
- Cigarette smoke (active or passive)
- Strong fumes or smells
- High atmospheric pollution levels
- Emotion or stress
- Hormonal factors (menstruation, pregnancy)

BOX 21.2   Steroid reversibility test

- Measure the PEF (best of three readings)
- Patient takes 30 mg prednisolone in the morning for 14 days
- Measure the PEF (best of three readings) on the 14th day

Alternatively, the patient can measure their PEF at home during the trial

---

BOX 21.3   Percentage change from baseline

$$\frac{\text{Post-test PEF} - \text{Pre-test PEF}}{\text{Pre-test PEF}} \times 100$$

---

basis of a test suitable for children or young adults accustomed to exercise. Facilities for the patient to exercise safely, under constant supervision, are necessary. Occasionally, significant bronchospasm can result, so a short-acting bronchodilator should be available. A fall of 20% and 60 l/min in the PEF following exercise is positive for asthma (Box 21.4).[3]

Serial PEF

Diurnal variability of PEF is characteristic of asthma. The patient records their PEF (best of three readings) first thing in the morning, before using any inhalers, and in the early evening, over a 2-week period. Results are recorded on a chart. A positive result is a variability of 20% and 60 l/min or more on at least 3 days over a 2-week period (Box 21.5).[3]

Diagnosis in young children

Children under 5 years old cannot use a PEF meter reliably. Some older children also have

problems. Here, diagnosis is based on the history and the response to asthma treatment. A symptom diary, recording relief bronchodilator use, nocturnal waking, ability to exercise and asthma symptoms, can be helpful.

TREATMENT OPTIONS

The goals of asthma treatment are:

- minimal symptoms day and night
- minimal need for reliever medication
- no exacerbations
- no limitation of physical activity
- normal lung function.[3]

For most asthma patients these aims are achievable with the correct treatment. Short-acting bronchodilators are used for quick symptom relief. Regular inhaled steroids to reduce underlying inflammation are needed for patients who have daily symptoms, nocturnal symptoms, abnormal lung function or acute attacks.

The drugs used to treat asthma can be broadly categorized into bronchodilators, to relieve

---

BOX 21.4   Exercise testing

- Measure the PEF (best of three readings)
- Get the patient to exercise vigorously for 6 minutes
- Take further PEF readings every 10 minutes for the next 30 minutes

---

BOX 21.5   Percentage variability in serial PEF (% amplitude best)

$$\frac{\text{Highest PEF} - \text{Lowest PEF}}{\text{Highest PEF}} \times 100$$

bronchospasm, and inhaled steroids and other anti-inflammatory treatments, to reduce inflammation in the airways, reducing BHR and preventing bronchospasm (Box 21.6).

Bronchodilators

There are three types of bronchodilator therapies used for asthma:

- *Beta$_2$ stimulant bronchodilators* are available as short- and long-acting inhaled therapies and as long-acting oral therapies. Short-acting inhaled beta$_2$ stimulants should be used 'as needed' by all patients with symptomatic asthma. Long-acting beta$_2$ stimulants are used twice daily in addition to inhaled steroids for patients inadequately controlled on inhaled steroids and short-acting beta$_2$ stimulants.
- *Anticholinergic bronchodilators* are available as short- and long-acting inhaled therapies. They are most often used for patients with severe asthma, or those with mixed asthma and chronic obstructive pulmonary disease, and are best used regularly, rather than 'as needed'.
- *Theophyllines* are long-acting, oral drugs. They are used infrequently nowadays, because they can cause nausea and also more serious side-effects such as seizures and cardiac arrhythmias.

Anti-inflammatory therapies

Inhaled steroids

These are the first-choice treatment for the prevention of asthma. Taken regularly inhaled steroids reduce symptoms and the risk of acute attacks. The inhaled steroids are usually used twice daily, although some are licensed for once-daily use at night in well-controlled asthma.

Unlike oral steroids they do not cause serious side-effects with long-term use in standard doses. Minor, local side-effects of oral candidiasis or hoarseness may occur, but can usually be resolved by changing the inhaler device.

Leukotriene receptor inhibitors

Leukotrienes are one of the inflammatory mediators of asthma. Two oral drugs, montelukast (Singular) and zafirlukast (Accolate), block the leukotriene receptor sites and have been found to be useful for some patients.

Oral steroids

Oral steroids are essential to aid life-saving in acute, severe asthma but are a last resort for maintenance treatment. A small minority of asthma patients, usually under specialist care,

---

BOX 21.6 Drug treatments for asthma

Bronchodilators
- Beta$_2$ stimulants
  - Short-acting: salbutamol, terbutaline
  - Long-acting: salmeterol, eformoterol
  - Oral: salbutamol
- Anticholinergics
  - Short-acting: ipratropium
  - Long-acting: oxitropium
- Theophyllines

Anti-inflammatory therapies
- Inhaled steroids:
  - beclometasone
  - budesonide
  - fluticasone
  - mometasone
- Leukotriene receptor antagonists:
  - montelukast
  - zafirlukast

Treatment for acute attacks
- High-dose inhaled beta$_2$ stimulants:
  - nebulized salbutamol or terbutaline, or 10–15 puffs of salbutamol terbutaline through a spacer may be equally effective
- Oral steroids:
  - prednisolone tablets
  - soluble prednisolone

require oral steroid treatment as well as high doses of inhaled steroids for maintenance.

In acute asthma oral steroids are given in short courses at high dose in the morning:

- age 2–5 years: 20 mg prednisolone for up to 3 days
- age 5–12 years: 30–40 mg prednisolone for up to 3 days
- adults: 40–50 mg prednisolone for at least 5 days or until recovery.

INHALERS

Inhaled therapy enables lower doses to be used, producing fewer side-effects. However, inhalers are more difficult to use than tablets and syrups and, because doses are small, correct technique is vital if the drug is to reach the airways.

You should familiarize yourself with the inhalers most commonly prescribed in your practice so that you can teach patients to use them and check inhaler technique. There are four main types of inhaler:

- pressurized metered dose inhalers (pMDIs)
- spacers
- breath-actuated pMDIs
- dry powder inhalers (DPIs).

pMDIs

These are the cheapest and most widely prescribed inhaler devices. They are also the most difficult to use correctly. The patient needs to be able precisely to coordinate actuation of the inhaler with inhalation.

Spacers

Spacers – or, to use a more correct term, holding chambers – remove the need to coordinate. The pMDI is actuated into the spacer from which the patient inhales deeply or takes 4–5 normal 'tidal' breaths through it.

Spacers improve drug delivery and reduce local inhaled steroid side-effects. They are the ideal method for delivering high-dose inhaled steroids at all ages and are the only method available for children under 5 years old.[4] Babies and toddlers need spacers with mask attachments. The drawback of spacers is their size, as they tend to be cumbersome and are not particularly portable.

Breath-actuated pMDIs

These release a dose of medication when the patient breathes in. They eliminate the need to coordinate and are easy to use. They are more expensive and not all therapies are available in this form.

Dry powder inhalers

These are also breath-actuated and, although some require more manual dexterity than others, most are easy and convenient. They allow the patient to see when the inhaler is running out or count the doses used. This is not possible with other inhalers.

ACUTE AND WORSENING ASTHMA

Worsening asthma is indicated by:

- increasing symptoms
- falling PEF or increasing diurnal variation in PEF
- increased need for short-acting beta$_2$ stimulants
- reduced effectiveness of short-acting beta$_2$ stimulants
- nocturnal disturbance with cough and wheeze
- decreasing exercise tolerance.

In a general practice setting it is important that you can recognize and accurately assess the severity of an asthma attack and that patients are taught to recognize when their asthma is getting out of control and when they need to seek help.

In the event of an acute asthma attack there should be a practice protocol and a patient group direction to enable you to initiate treatment promptly. See Box 21.7 for features of acute asthma. Severe attacks require immediate treatment and, in the case of life-threatening asthma, rapid transfer to hospital by ambulance.

PATIENT EDUCATION

All patients need to be taught how to use their inhalers and need to understand what their treatments are for. Some will want more detailed information. Some will understand complex medical information, but for others such detail will be confusing.

Information must be given in language that is meaningful to patients and be individually tailored and personalized (Box 21.8). It is most effective when given in small, regularly repeated amounts. Written information is helpful reinforcement. High-quality, independent patient information is available from the National Asthma Campaign. All patients should have a written personalized asthma action plan, to enable them to recognize and adjust their treatment to cope with worsening asthma.[3]

It is important that patients understand when to seek urgent medical help. Such information is most effective when it is written down and personalized. Asthma deaths are frequently related to delays in seeking help and delays in commencing appropriate therapy. Any of the following indicate a severe attack:

- difficulty in speaking because of breathlessness
- severe breathlessness on minimal exertion or at rest
- a need to use a short-acting bronchodilator inhaler more than every 4 hours and/or failure to get complete relief from the inhaler
- a PEF reading that is less than 50% of the patient's usual best.

BOX 21.7 Features of acute asthma

Mild attack: PEF > 75% best
- *Pulse rate*: normal
- *Respiratory rate*: normal
- *Ability to talk/feed*: normal
- *Colour*: normal

Moderate attack: PEF 50–75% best
- *Pulse rate*:
  < 110/min (adults)
  < 120/min (5–12 years)
  < 130/min (2–5 years)
- *Respiratory rate*:
  < 25/min (adults)
  < 30/min (5–12 years)
  < 50/min (2–5 years)
- *Ability to talk/feed*: normal
- *Colour*: normal

Severe attack: PEF 33–50% best
- *Pulse rate*:
  > 110/min (adults)
  > 120/min (5–12 years)
  > 130/min (2–5 years)
- *Respiratory rate*:
  > 25/min (adults)
  > 30/min (5–12 years)
  > 50/min (2–5 years)
- *Ability to talk/feed*: unable to complete a sentence in one breath/unable to feed
- *Colour*: normal

Life-threatening attack: PEF < 33%
- *Any of these signs in a severe attack*:
  - pallor or cyanosis
  - feeble respiratory effort
  - 'silent' chest
  - bradycardia, arrhythmia or hypotension
  - restlessness/agitation or altered consciousness

Often patients are concerned about exceeding the stated dose of their short-acting bronchodilator. In an emergency situation they can be reassured that it is safe (and may be life-saving) for them to take repeated doses while they are waiting for help. In the acute situation 10–15 doses through a spacer (one puff at a time) is as effective as one dose via a nebulizer.

Although it may cause tremor and palpitations it is usually well tolerated. If patients have an asthma action plan that includes an emergency supply of oral steroids they should be told to take the first dose immediately.

BOX 21.8   National Respiratory Training Centre criteria for structured asthma care

Minimal involvement (no formal training)

1. Compile asthma register
2. Take structured history
3. Take peak flow readings in surgery
4. Teach how to use peak flow meter at home and how to chart a diary card
5. Demonstrate instruct and check inhaler technique

Medium involvement (basic training)

Activities 1–5 plus:

6. Carry out diagnostic procedures (e.g. reversibility, exercise and serial PEF readings)
7. Improve asthma education
8. Provide explanatory literature
9. Spot poor control, with referral back to GP
10. Establish regular follow-up procedures

Maximum involvement (with experience and more advanced training)

Activities 1–10 plus:

11. Carry out full assessment and regular follow-up
12. Formulate structured action plan in conjunction with GP and patient
13. Prepare prescription for GP's signature
14. Give telephone advice/additional appointments where appropriate
15. See patients first in an emergency

CONCLUSION

Asthma can seriously disrupt patients' lives and still causes 15,000 deaths each year. Appropriately trained practice nurses can improve the lives of asthma patients and gain enormous job satisfaction while doing so.

ESSENTIAL SKILLS

- Understanding of the mechanisms of asthma and the diagnostic techniques
- Familiarity with BTS/SIGN Guidelines
- Ability to teach and check correct inhaler technique
- Ability to take accurate PEF readings in the surgery
- Ability to teach a patient how to chart serial PEF readings at home
- Ability to accurately assess the severity of an asthma attack
- Ability to initiate appropriate management in the event of an acute or life-threatening asthma attack
- Ability to provide up-to-date patient information

REFERENCES

1. National Heart Lung and Blood Institute. National Institutes of Health international consensus report on the diagnosis and treatment of asthma. Eur Resp J 1992; 5: 601–641.
2. National Asthma Campaign. Out in the open: a true picture of asthma in the United Kingdom today. Asthma J 2001; 6(3 Suppl).
3. British Thoracic Society, Scottish Intercollegiate Guidelines Network. British guideline on the management of asthma. Thorax 2003; 58(Suppl 1): i1–i94.

4. National Institute for Health and Clinical Excellence. Guidance on the Use of Inhaler Systems (Devices) in Children under the Age of 5 years with Chronic Asthma. Technology Appraisal Guidelines No. 10. London: NICE, 2000.

FURTHER READING

National Respiratory Training Centre. Simply Asthma: A Practical Pocket Book. Warwick: NRTC. For contact details see below.

USEFUL WEBSITES

Charts of the BTS and SIGN guidelines are available at: http://www.brit-thoracic.org.uk

Guidance on inhaler devices for children is available at: http://www.nice.org.uk

National Asthma Campaign Helpline provides patient information: Tel. 0845 701 0203; http:// www.asthma.org.uk

National Respiratory Training Centre: Tel. 01926 493313; http:// www.nrtc.org.uk

Respiratory Education and Training Centre: http://www.respiratoryetc.com

Chapter 22

COPD management

Rachel Booker

Chronic obstructive pulmonary disease (COPD) is characterized by airflow limitation that is progressive, not fully reversible and associated with an abnormal inflammatory response to noxious particles or gases.[1] The term is used to embrace a spectrum of conditions including emphysema, chronic bronchitis and some cases of chronic asthma.

In the UK, COPD is responsible for an annual toll of 30,000 deaths, which usually follow an extended period of disability, dependency and increasing use of health service resources.[2] However, there is still a considerable amount that can be done for patients. Appropriate management can improve symptoms and quality of life.

RISK FACTORS AND PRESENTATION

COPD is overwhelmingly a smoking-related condition, although 10–15% of cases occur in non-smokers – mainly for occupational reasons. A smoking history of more than 20 pack-years is considered to be significant – a pack-year being the number of cigarettes smoked daily divided by 20 and multiplied by the number of years for which the patient has been a smoker.[1, 3]

About 15–20% of smokers experience an accelerated decline in their lung function.[4] Unfortunately, the process is slowly and insidiously progressive, so COPD symptoms do not become apparent until about half of the respiratory reserve is irretrievably lost. Late presentation is common.

COPD causes progressive breathlessness on exertion. Cough and sputum production are also common and some patients complain of wheeze and 'tightness' in the chest. A 'smoker's cough' may be an early warning sign of early, presymptomatic COPD, and such patients may be considered for screening with spirometry.[1]

COPD shares many of the features of asthma and the two conditions are often confused. Long-standing, chronic asthma can also lead to irreversible airflow obstruction and be indistinguishable from smoking-related COPD. The key differences are highlighted in Table 22.1.

DIAGNOSIS

The diagnosis of COPD relies on the clinical history, supported by objective tests of lung function and a 4–6 week trial of bronchodilator therapy. Spirometry is the recommended diagnostic method.[1, 3] However, poorly performed spirometry is useless. If you are required to use a spirometer you must be trained and proficient in its use.

A spirometer measures:

- forced vital capacity (FVC) – the volume of air exhaled forcibly from maximum inhalation to maximum exhalation

- forced expired volume in one second (FEV_1) – the volume of air exhaled in the first second of a forced blow from maximum inhalation
- the ratio of FEV_1 to FVC (FEV_1/FVC, FEV_1% or FER).

Tests of the efficacy of bronchodilators and corticosteroids, conducted in a clinically stable patient, help to confirm whether or not the airflow obstruction is reversible (Box 22.1). However, routine reversibility testing for diagnoses of COPD is no longer recommended. If the FEV_1 improves by more than 400 ml the reversibility test is positive, suggesting an asthmatic element in the condition. Lung function that reverses to within normal limits is not compatible with a diagnosis of COPD.

Spirometry readings compatible with a diagnosis of COPD are:

- FEV_1/FVC < 70%
- FEV_1 < 80% of the predicted value.

FEV_1 is used to classify disease severity (Box 22.2).[3] The levels of severity have been brought into line with international guidelines.

Middle-aged smokers have a high incidence of conditions such as ischaemic heart disease and lung cancer, as well as being susceptible to COPD. Comorbidity can cause diagnostic confusion and complicate management, so it is important to exclude alternative causes for symptoms before applying the diagnostic label of COPD.

TABLE 22.1 Symptoms and presentation of COPD and asthma		
Feature	COPD	Asthma
Onset	Age 45 years and over	Any age; childhood most common
Smoking history	Usually 20 pack-years or more	May or may not be a smoker
Symptoms	Slowly progressive shortness of breath on exertion; morning cough and sputum	Nocturnal cough and wheeze; shortness of breath on exertion
Variability of symptoms	Little day-to-day variability	Good days and bad days
Previous/family history	No history of atopy or asthma; may or may not be family history of COPD	Often a positive family and/or personal history of asthma or atopic disease

Close teamwork with medical colleagues is essential, and patients should be referred for a specialist opinion if there are any grounds for doubt.

DRUG TREATMENT

Choice of drugs or drug combinations should be decided individually. The therapeutic response is assessed in terms of improved symptoms – less breathlessness, improved walking distance, improved well-being – rather than improvements in lung function.

Bronchodilators

Bronchodilators are the mainstay of COPD treatment. Patients do experience reduced symptoms, even though their reduced lung function is irreversible. Both short- and long-acting beta$_2$ agonist and anticholinergic bronchodilators are beneficial (Box 22.3).

Inhaled bronchodilators work more quickly and cause fewer side-effects than tablets. COPD patients may need higher doses than are used in asthma, and can be reassured that the drugs are safe for regular use. There is no benefit in doing without them. Users do not become addicted, and the drugs do not lose their effect with repeated use.

BOX 22.1   Reversibility tests

Beta$_2$ agonist
- Use salbutamol (Ventolin) 5 mg via a nebulizer or four puffs via a metered dose inhaler (MDI) and spacer
- Retest after 15 minutes

Anticholinergics
- Use ipratropium bromide (Atrovent) 250–500 μg via a nebulizer or four puffs via an MDI and spacer
- Retest after 30–45 minutes

Combined treatment
- Use salbutamol 2.5 mg plus ipratropium bromide (Combivent) 500 μg via a nebulizer or four puffs via an MDI and spacer
- Retest after 30–45 minutes

Corticosteroids
- Record post-bronchodilator spirometry at the start and end of the test
- Oral test: use prednisolone 30–40 mg in the morning for 2 weeks
- Inhaled test: use beclomethasone 1000 μg, or budesonide (Pulmicort) 800 μg, or fluticasone (Flixotide) 500 μg daily for 6–12 weeks

---

BOX 22.2   Classification of disease severity

COPD severity	FEV$_1$ (% predicted)
Mild	50–80
Moderate	30–49
Severe	< 30

BOX 22.3   Bronchodilators for COPD

Beta$_2$ agonists
- Short-acting:
  - salbutamol (Ventolin)
  - terbutaline (Bricanyl)
- Long-acting:
  - salmeterol (Serevent)

Anticholinergics
- Short-acting:
  - ipratropium bromide (Atrovent)
- Long-acting:
  - oxitropium bromide (Oxivent)
  - tiotropium (Spiriva)

Combined treatment
- Salbutamol + ipratropium bromide (Combivent)
- Fluticasone + salmeterol (Seretide)
- Budesonide + eformoterol (Symbicont)

Theophyllines may be helpful in more difficult cases, but problematic side-effects and drug interactions reduce their usefulness.

Corticosteroids

In asthma, corticosteroids reduce symptoms and the risk of acute attacks and restore lung function. In smoking-related COPD, neither inhaled nor oral corticosteroids produce significant improvements in lung function at any stage of the disease.

None of the national or international COPD guidelines recommends long-term oral cortico-steroid use in COPD, because of the significant risk of serious side-effects. Current British guidelines recommend inhaled corticosteroids only for patients with a positive corticosteroid reversibility test.[3] However, it has been shown that inhaled corticosteroids reduce the frequency of exacerbations and slow the decline in health status of patients with severe disease.[5]

Recent international COPD guidelines recommend inhaled corticosteroids for patients who suffer frequent exacerbations and have FEV_1 measures less than 50% of the predicted level.[1]

New British COPD guidelines were published in February 2004 (see http://www.nice.org.uk).

Combination therapy

Inhalers containing both a long-acting $beta_2$ agonist and a corticosteroid are now available. Formulations of budesonide plus eformoterol (Symbicort), and fluticasone plus salmeterol (Seretide) are licensed for use in COPD. Both combinations can reduce exacerbation frequency and improve lung function, symptoms and health status in severe COPD.[6, 7]

Inhaler choice

When choosing an inhaler, the same consider-ations apply to both COPD and asthma. Patients need to be able to use the device and it should be acceptable and fit in to their lifestyle.

Metered-dose inhalers (MDIs) with spacers are useful, but are not very portable and may restrict the patient's willingness to get out and socialize.

Regular nebulized bronchodilators are helpful for a small number of patients, but assessment by a specialist is needed before home nebulizers are recommended.[8] Repeated dosing from a hand-held inhaler may be just as effective and is a cheaper, more convenient option.

You should be familiar with the types of inhaler commonly used in your practice and be able to teach and check inhaler technique.

Management of exacerbations

Most COPD patients experience periodic worsening of their condition. The first-line treatment in an exacerbation is to increase the dose or frequency of the bronchodilator. Nebulizers are not usually necessary.

Antibiotics are needed if the patient has an increase in any two of the classic symptoms – sputum production, sputum purulence and breath-lessness.[1, 3] Patients should be advised to contact their doctor promptly in such circumstances.

A short course of oral corticosteroids (7–10 days prednisolone 30–40 mg), with or without antibiotics, can shorten the exacerbation and is usually given if the patient fails to respond to an increase in bronchodilators alone.

NON-DRUG APPROACHES

Smoking cessation

Smoking cessation is the only intervention that slows the rate of lung-function decline and must be actively encouraged in all patients with COPD. If the patient does stop smoking, the rate of lung function decline returns to that of a non-smoker or non-susceptible smoker.

The key messages are:

- it is never too late to stop smoking.
- the earlier you stop the better.

Nicotine replacement therapy and bupropion (Zyban) are both effective, and patients should be advised to use them.[9] Brief intervention and advice from you can help, but patients who experience difficulty may need to be referred to a specialist smoking-cessation adviser.

Pulmonary rehabilitation

Breathlessness on exertion engenders panic, resulting in anxiety and activity avoidance. The patient then becomes less and less physically fit, more and more breathless, socially isolated, depressed and dependent. Pulmonary rehabilitation is a programme of exercise and education that aims to break this vicious cycle.

Regular, supervised exercise over several weeks, combined with structured education, is extremely effective. Patients make less use of healthcare resources and achieve significant improvements in disability and quality of life.

Unfortunately, the provision of pulmonary rehabilitation services remains patchy at best. Where services are not available patients should be encouraged to exercise regularly, within their capability, and to keep as active as possible for as long as possible.

Remember, breathlessness is not harmful. Positive encouragement, reassurance and education about the disease and how to manage it can be helpful.

Influenza vaccination

Annual influenza vaccination should be actively encouraged. It can reduce the risk of serious illness and death by about 50%.[10]

Nutrition

Patients should be encouraged to eat a healthy diet, rich in fresh fruit and vegetables. COPD patients are often malnourished. It is difficult to shop, cook and eat if you are breathless, and weight loss is associated with a worsening prognosis.

Underweight patients can be encouraged to eat small, frequent, high-calorie, easily prepared meals, but may still need to be referred to a dietitian. At the other extreme, obesity increases breathlessness, so some patients may need advice on weight reduction.

CONCLUSION

Managing COPD patients can be challenging, but also extremely rewarding. A positive approach from you, coupled with advice about lifestyle, exercise and the appropriate use of drugs, can help patients and their families to cope and make the most of life with COPD.

ESSENTIAL SKILLS

- Learn the clinical signs differentiating asthma and COPD
- Find out about spirometry training through your practice or PCT
- Work as a team with medical colleagues and refer patients for a specialist opinion if there are any grounds for doubt
- Read the new NICE guidance on COPD (available at http://www.nice.org.uk)

REFERENCES

1. National Institutes of Health. National Heart Lung and Blood Institute. Global Initiative For Chronic Obstructive Lung Disease. 2003. Available at: http://www.goldcopd.com/revised_es.pdf

2. British Thoracic Society. The burden of lung disease: a statistics report for the British Thoracic Society. London: BTS, 2001. Available at: http://www.brit-thoracic.org.uk/docs/BurdenofLungDisease.pdf

3. British Thoracic Society. BTS guidelines for the management of chronic obstructive pulmonary disease. Thorax 1997; 52(Suppl 5): S1–S28. Available at: http://www.brit-thoracic.org.uk/docs/COPDtext.pdf

4. Fletcher C, Peto R. The natural history of chronic airflow obstruction. BMJ 1977; 1(6077): 1645–1648.

5. Burge PS, Calverley PM, Jones PW, et al. Randomised double-blind placebo controlled study of fluticasone propionate in patients with moderate to severe chronic obstructive pulmonary disease: the ISOLDE trial. BMJ 2000; 320(7245): 1297–1303.

6. Calverley P, Pauwels R, Vestbo J, et al. Combined salmeterol and fluticasone in the treatment of chronic obstructive pulmonary disease: a randomised controlled trial. Lancet 2003; 361(9356): 449–456.

7. Szafranski W, Cukier A, Ramirez A, et al. Efficacy and safety of budesonide formoterol in the management of chronic obstructive pulmonary disease. Eur Resp J 2003; 21(1): 74–81.

8. British Thoracic Society. Current best practice for nebuliser treatment. Thorax 1997; 52(Suppl 2): S1–S3.

9. National Institute for Health and Clinical Excellence. Guidance on the Use of Nicotine Replacement Therapy and Bupropion for Smoking Cessation. Technology Appraisal Guidance 39. London: NICE, 2002.

10. Nichol KL, Margolis KL, Wuorenma J, et al. The efficacy and cost effectiveness of vaccination against influenza among elderly persons living in the community. N Engl J Med 1994; 331: 778–784.

USEFUL WEBSITES

National Respiratory Training Centre: runs one-day essential skills training in spirometry and COPD and distance-learning and degree-level modules accredited with the Open University. Produces a pocket book *Simply COPD* and a CD-ROM on respiratory therapeutics, including inhaler techniques. The Athenaeum, 10 Church Street, Warwick CV34 4AB; Tel. 01926 493313; e-mail: enquiries@nrtc.org.uk; http://www.nrtc.org.uk

British Thoracic Society COPD Consortium: for information on COPD and a booklet on spirometry. http://www.brit-thoracic.org.uk/copd

Respiratory Education and Training Centre: for training in COPD and spirometry. http://www.respiratoryetc.com

Section 3

Health maintenance and clinical procedures

SECTION CONTENTS

Chapter 23

12-Lead ECG recording

Nicola Stevens

An essential skill for most practice nurses is 12-lead electrocardiogram (ECG) recording. It should be borne in mind that in commencing any new role you are accountable for your own professional practice and must ensure that you learn and understand the appropriate theory to underpin new practical skills, in order to enhance patient care.[1,2] Supervision of a newly acquired skill is also needed, and you will need to investigate the training and supervision available locally before agreeing to start a new role.

NORMAL CONDUCTION OF THE HEART

The sinoatrial (SA) node initiates an impulse causing depolarization (contraction), which spreads through the atria and is represented on an ECG by the P wave. The SA node also controls the pace of the heart – usually 70–80 beats per minute. Depolarization continues to the atrioventricular (AV) node, with the electrical discharge passing quickly through the bundle of His, which then divides into right and left branches. Conduction then continues via the Purkinje fibres, which allows contraction of the ventricles.

The main waves on an ECG are P, Q, R, S and T. They represent electrical discharging (depolarization, causing contraction) or electrical recharging (repolarization, causing relaxation) (Figure 23.1).

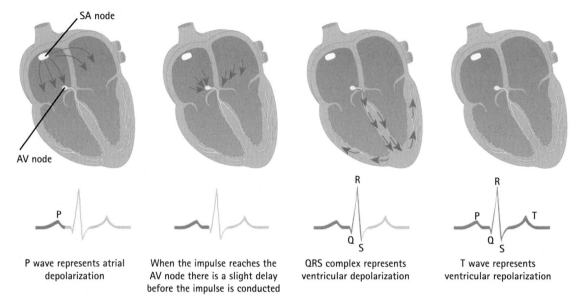

P wave represents atrial depolarization

When the impulse reaches the AV node there is a slight delay before the impulse is conducted

QRS complex represents ventricular depolarization

T wave represents ventricular repolarization

Figure 23.1   Conduction pathways.

NORMAL 12-LEAD ECG RECORDING

An ECG is an assessment tool to be used in conjunction with other assessments, for example the patient history. It can provide evidence to support a diagnosis.

ECG is a simple, non-invasive investigation recording electrical activity of the heart from 12 different leads or viewpoints, via the 10 electrodes placed on the patient. The size of each wave on the ECG recording corresponds to the electrical voltage generated (measured in millivolts). The paper grid to measure these viewpoints measures time (horizontally) and voltage (vertically) (Figure 23.2). Each small box horizontally represents 0.04 seconds and each large box 0.20 seconds.

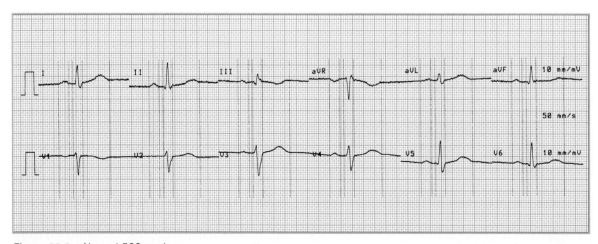

Figure 23.2   Normal ECG tracing.

Normally, ECGs are recorded at a speed of 25 mm/s and a sensitivity of 10 mm/mV. Any variations to this should be clearly identified on the recording to avoid misinterpretation. All 12 leads/viewpoints will be recorded on a full-page layout (multichannel recorder) or sequentially (single-channel recorder).

EQUIPMENT

The range of recorders available is enormous.[3] Purchasing decisions need to take account of:

- price
- reliability
- portability
- ease of use
- servicing
- performance characteristics.

Hospital-based medical physics departments can help with choosing an appropriate machine that adheres to Medical Devices Agency Standards.[4]

PATIENT PREPARATION

The patient should have the procedure explained to them along with the indication (Box 23.1). Emphasis should be placed on the non-invasive nature of the test. The patient should lie flat on the

---

BOX 23.1   Indications for ECG recording

- Chest pain
- Suspected myocardial infarction
- Suspected cardiac anomaly
- Suspected cardiac arrhythmia
- Pre-employment medical
- Pre-surgery assessment
- Chronic disease management
- Some drug treatments

---

examination couch with a pillow, be comfortable, relaxed and warm (shivering produces muscle tremor, which interferes with the tracing). Privacy should also be ensured. There is usually no need to remove jewellery such as watches unless tracing problems occur. Tights may be worn as long as there are no contact problems. Bras should be removed for correct chest electrode placement and a blanket or sheet placed over the patient to provide privacy and warmth.

A variety of electrodes is available: chest suction cups and limb plates, or self-adhesive electrodes, which require little or no skin preparation. Dry skin or perspiration can be simply removed with a dry swab. Alcohol-impregnated wipes are not required. Partial shaving is only required in particularly hairy individuals where electrode contact is problematic.

ELECTRODE POSITIONING

Each lead looks at a specific surface of the heart, and therefore correct positioning of electrodes is essential to obtain a diagnostically useful recording. By attaching electrodes to the right arm, left arm and left leg, three major planes for detecting electrical activity can be recorded. These three planes form a hypothetical triangle (Einthoven's triangle) with the heart in the middle. A fourth electrode is attached to the left leg, but serves only as an earth and is not used for recording purposes.

The chest electrodes V1, V2, V3, V4, V5 and V6 are attached as shown in Figure 23.3:

- V1 – fourth intercostal space to the right of the sternum
- V2 – fourth intercostal space to the left of the sternum
- skip to V4 – fifth intercostal space in the midclavicular line
- V3 – halfway between V2 and V4
- V5 – fifth intercostal space at the anterior axillary line

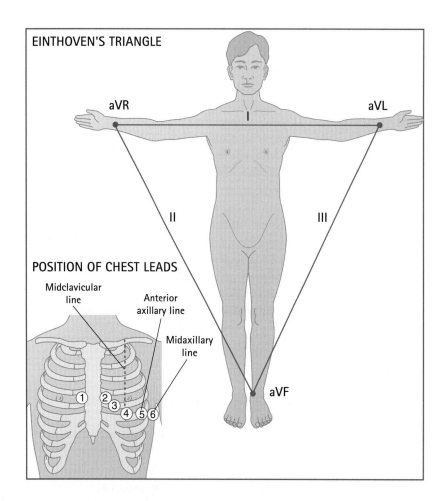

EINTHOVEN'S TRIANGLE

aVR   I   aVL

II   III

POSITION OF CHEST LEADS

Midclavicular line

Anterior axillary line

Midaxillary line

① ② ③ ④ ⑤ ⑥

aVF

Figure 23.3 Electrode positions for 12-lead ECG recording.

- V6 – fifth intercostal space at the midaxillary line.

Familiarize yourself with the local equipment available – a manual should be available to refer to for machine operation. It is also important to know how to change the recording paper, charge the machine, servicing arrangements, where supplies of electrodes/paper are kept and how to order further supplies. A practical demonstration should initially be offered by an appropriately trained professional, such as a GP, experienced practice nurse or trainer. Supervised practice should then be instigated until skill is mastered competently. The patient should be made comfortable after the test and made aware of the results procedure.

The recording should be labelled with the patient's name, date of birth, and date and time of test. Any symptoms experienced during the test, such as chest pain, should also be documented on

ESSENTIAL SKILLS

- Explain the indication to patients
- Service equipment regularly
- Prepare patients appropriately and position electrodes correctly
- Eliminate tracing problems
- Ask a doctor to review recording and document result

BOX 23.2   The recording

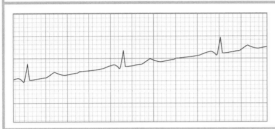

WANDERING BASELINE

Cause: Poor electrode contact, heavy respiration or restless patient

Solution: Check electrode placement for good contact, reassure patient and advise to breathe normally, lie still and not to talk while recording

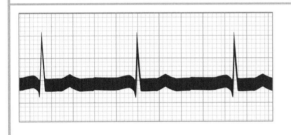

SOMATIC (MUSCLE) TREMOR

Cause: Skeletal muscle tension

Solution: Reassure patient to relax, ensure privacy, warmth, procedure explained adequately

AC INTERFERENCE

Cause: Electrical equipment in vicinity of patient, or defective recorder

Solution: Move electrical equipment adjacent to patient, service equipment as manufacturer advises, if recorder fault is suspected send for inspection and repair

the recording. An ECG recording is not validated until reviewed by a doctor at an appropriate time. Should any abnormalities be suspected or symptoms experienced during the test the recording should be reviewed while the patient remains in the surgery. Computer-based interpretation offered on some recorders also needs a doctor to validate the result.

COMMON TRACING PROBLEMS

Often recorders incorporate filters that help reduce the effects of interference.

REFERENCES

1. United Kingdom Central Council for Nursing Midwifery and Health Visiting. The Scope of Professional Practice. London: UKCC, 1992.
2. Nursing and Midwifery Council. Code of Professional Practice. London: NMC, 2002.
3. Johnston K. The use of ECGs to record heart activity. Professional Nurse 1999; 14(6): 417–423.
4. Medical Devices Agency. Medical Device and Equipment Management for Hospital and Community-Based Organisations. Device Bulletin, DB 9801. London: MDA, 1998.

FURTHER READING

Bayer MJ. Need to Know ECG Facts. London: Lippincott, 1995.

Chernecky C, et al. ECGs and the Heart. Philadelphia: Saunders, 2002.

Garcia TB, Holtz NE. Introduction to 12 Lead ECG: the Art of Interpretation. London: Jones & Bartlett, 2003.

Hampton JR. The ECG Made Easy. New York: Churchill Livingstone, 1997.

Houghton AR, Gray YD. Making Sense of ECG. London: Arnold, 1998.

Chapter 24

Ear examination and management

Hilary Harkin

CHAPTER CONTENTS

Basic ear care involves carrying out examinations (Boxes 24.1 and 24.2), understanding the implications of the results and providing relevant health education for patients. Ear irrigation is covered in Chapter 25. In order to provide this service you need to have an understanding of the anatomy and physiology of the ear. Information on the ear can be downloaded free of charge from the ENT nursing website (see Useful Websites). Educating patients to care for their ears reduces the chance of infection and wax impaction, and has the

---

BOX 24.1   Ear examinations

A routine ear examination should be carried out:

- for all adult patients (> 16 years old) new to the practice
- at annual checks on patients over the age of 65 years who wear hearing aids
- at annual checks on patients who have required wax removal (irrigation, manual removal, microsuction) in the past
- for patients presenting with ear-related symptoms (hearing loss, discharge, pain, vertigo, tinnitus, itching, blocked feeling/fullness in the ear)
- for patients having problems with hearing aids (i.e. whistling) or patients over the age of 60 years with an audiology appointment

added benefit of reducing our workload as practice nurses.

Most nurses performing ear syringing from general practice have been taught using a 'see one, do one' method.[1] This poor practice is perpetuated by experienced nurses teaching this method to new recruits. An ideal way to break this cycle is to target new practice nurses and recommend attendance on a recognized ear care study day.

The updated and improved ear care they are taught can then be shared with colleagues.

MANAGEMENT OF WAX

If the result of the examination is wax in the ear canal then it should be assessed for colour,

---

BOX 24.2   Guidance for ear examination

1. Before careful physical examination of the ear, listen to the patient, elicit symptoms and take a careful history. Explain each step of any procedure or examination and ensure that the patient understands and gives consent. Ensure that both you and the patient are seated comfortably, at the same level, and that you have privacy.

2. Turn on the otoscope and use the light to examine the pinna, outer canal and adjacent scalp. Check for previous surgery incision scars, infection, discharge, swelling and signs of skin lesions or defects. Decide on the most appropriate sized speculum that will fit comfortably into the ear and place it on the otoscope.

3. Gently pull the pinna upwards and outwards to straighten the ear canal (directly down and back in children). Bear in mind that localized infection or inflammation will cause this procedure to be painful. If such an infection is present, do not continue.

4. Holding the otoscope like a pen, rest your little finger on the patient's head to detect any unexpected movement. Use the light to observe the direction of the ear canal and the tympanic membrane. Visualization of the eardrum can usually be improved by using the left hand for the left ear and the right hand for the right ear, but use your own judgement. Insert the speculum gently into the canal to pass through the hairs at the entrance to the canal.

5. Looking through the otoscope check the ear canal and tympanic membrane. The ear cannot be judged to be normal until all the areas of the membrane are viewed. Adjust your head and the otoscope to ensure that you can see the light reflex, handle of malleus, pars flaccida, pars tensa and anterior recess. If your view of the tympanic membrane is hampered by the presence of wax, then wax removal will have to be carried out. Figure 24.1 shows an otoscopic view of a normal healthy ear.

6. Carefully check the condition of the skin in the ear canal as you withdraw the otoscope. If there is doubt about the patient's hearing an audiological assessment should be made. Providing they meet the criteria stated in local referral guidelines, older adults with a bilateral hearing loss can be referred directly to the audiology department.

7. Document what you observed in both ears, the procedure carried out, the condition of the tympanic membrane and external auditory meatus and treatment given. Findings should be recorded following the Nursing and Midwifery Council (NMC) guidelines on record keeping and accountability. If any abnormality is found a referral should be made to the ENT outpatient department following local policy.

consistency, odour and location. If it is not reflecting the light of the otoscope and is dull and dark in colour then it tends to be harder.

As the otoscope magnifies, the amount of wax appears greater and it is often difficult to judge how far down the ear canal it is located. If there are hairs around the wax and it can be viewed with the headlight then it tends to be in the outer third. This wax can be removed manually by a competent practitioner.

Instruct the patient according to your clinical judgement on how to soften wax. A possible treatment could be to insert one drop of olive oil twice daily (morning and evening) into the ear(s) for one week prior to the appointment. If you explain that using olive oil can result in irrigation not taking so long, less discomfort and greater chance of success then patient compliance tends to be better. The patient can then return for irrigating or further instrumentation. Excessive soft wax or crumbly wax and debris can be irrigated or wiped out with cotton wool wound onto a Jobson Horne probe.

GUIDANCE FOR AURAL TOILET

Aural toilet is used to clear the ear canal of debris, discharge, soft wax or excess fluid following irrigation. This procedure should be taught on a recognized ear care study day where there is the opportunity to practise on a dummy head.

An individual assessment should be made of every patient to ensure that it is appropriate for aural toilet to be carried out.

The following guidelines form part of the NHS Modernisation Agency Guidance in Ear Care document. The entire document can be downloaded from the website (see Useful Websites):

- Examine the ear with an otoscope following the above guidance.
- Use a Jobson Horne probe and a small piece of fluffed up cotton wool, the size of a postage stamp, applied to the probe. Under direct vision

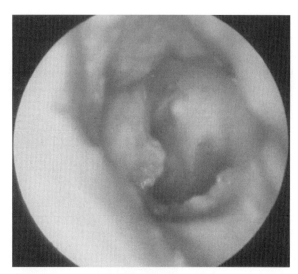

Figure 24.1   Normal otoscopic view of the ear.

(with headlight or head mirror and light) and pulling the pinna to straighten the canal, clean the ear canal with a gentle rotary action of the probe. Do not touch the tympanic membrane.
- Replace the cotton wool directly it becomes soiled.
- Re-examine the meatus intermittently, using the otoscope, during cleaning to check for any debris, discharge or crusts that remain in the canal at awkward angles.
- Give advice regarding ear care and document the procedure (Box 24.3).

HOW TO ADMINISTER OLIVE OIL

Prior to prescribing it is essential to consider whether the patient will manage to administer their own ear drops or will require support from district nurses or a relative.

Recommend that the patient use a glass dropper bottle filled with olive oil. This can be purchased from a chemist, or if they have used previous wax dissolving drops they can wash out the glass bottle and insert olive oil into the clean container (almond oil or coconut oil could be used if the patient does not have a nut allergy).

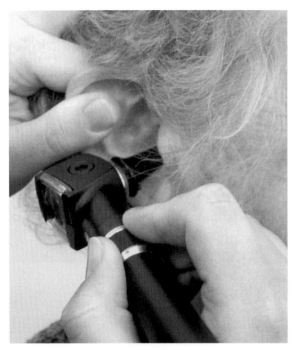

Figure 24.2   Ear examination.

I provide the patient with the following written information on how to instil olive oil (this can be downloaded from the ENT nursing website; see Useful Websites):

1. Insert the closed glass dropper bottle containing the oil into a cup of warm water for 2 minutes. Dry the container and insert one drop of oil onto your hand to ensure that it is not too hot. If you feel the oil is too hot wait for it to cool prior to commencing.
2. Holding the prepared glass dropper bottle lie on a bed, with the affected ear towards the ceiling.
3. With one hand pull the top of your ear upwards and outwards to straighten the ear canal.
4. Place the filled dropper part of the bottle of oil over the entrance to your ear canal and squeeze the dropper until one drop (or the amount specified by your nurse) is instilled. Maintain that position for 5 minutes. Wipe the excess drops that pool outside the ear when you sit up.

BOX 24.3   Advice to give to patients

- The ear canal is self-cleaning. To clean the outside of the ear use a damp flannel around and behind the ear after showering or bathing and a clean tissue to dry. Do not insert any implements such as cotton buds into the ear. They will damage the delicate skin lining the ear and increase the chance of you developing an ear infection, itchy ears or a problem with wax
- If the inside of your ear canal is very itchy you could try one drop of olive oil when itchy or with the frequency recommended by your nurse
- Try to prevent water entering the ears, as shampoos and soaps may irritate the skin
- If the entrance to the ear canal is very dry apply a skin moisturizing ointment twice daily. If you have experienced an external ear infection keep the ears dry
- Use cotton wool coated in petroleum jelly placed at the entrance to both ear canals or ear plugs to prevent water getting in the ears

ESSENTIAL SKILLS

- An understanding of the anatomy and physiology of the ear and ability to apply this to patient education
- The ability to carry out an ear examination using an otoscope
- The ability to recognize a normal tympanic membrane
- The ability to assess wax/debris in the ear canal and understand the options for removal
- Familiarity with the referral process for patients with problems related to the ear and/or hearing

Do not insert cotton wool, as this will absorb the drops.

5. If the drops are to be inserted into both ears repeat steps two to four on the other side.

EDUCATION AND TRAINING

Before practising ear care it is strongly recommended that you attend a recognized study day – speak to your practice development nurse or the training department at your primary care group or primary care trust.

Developing your understanding of the various ear problems frequently encountered in practice will enhance your ability to provide appropriate care. You should be able to identify the patients with conditions that you can treat and those who need to be referred to an ENT clinic.

REFERENCES

1. Rodgers R. Understanding the legalities of ear syringing. Practice Nurse 2000; 19(4): 166–169.

FURTHER READING

Harkin H. Evidence based ear care. Primary Health Care 2000; 10(8): 25–30.

Harkin H. Ear care guide unveiled. Primary Health Care 2002; 12(9): 20.

Price J. Problems of ear syringing. Practice Nurse 1997; 14(2):126–127.

USEFUL WEBSITES

ENT nursing website: the site includes guidance on the anatomy and physiology of the ear, advice on the insertion of drops and on care of the ears post-irrigation. Information is free to download. http://www.entnursing.com

NHS Modernisation Agency: management of ear care is covered in detail in the Action on ENT Steering Board's Ear Care Guidance Document which can be downloaded free, http://www.modern.nhs.uk, http://www.entnursing.com

Royal National Institute for the Deaf (RNID): produces a series of leaflets available to view or print, including one titled *Look After Your Ears*. http://www.rnid.org.uk

Chapter 25

Ear irrigation

Hilary Harkin

In Chapter 24 we looked at ear examination and general management. Now we turn our attention to ear irrigation.

Even if the patient has been referred by the GP, the ear should be examined to ensure the procedure is necessary and there are no abnormalities. The nurse performing the procedure needs to establish for himself or herself that manual removal is not appropriate for the wax/debris and that there are no contraindications to irrigation (see Chapter 24).

The procedure should always be referred to as 'irrigation', as the term syringing implies the use of a metal syringe to remove wax by the pressure of water. This method is dangerous to the patient and has resulted in litigation cases.[1] Computer-held records need to be altered to reflect the use of the electronic irrigator.

GUIDANCE FOR EAR IRRIGATION USING THE ELECTRONIC IRRIGATOR

The guidelines in Box 25.1 form part of the NHS Modernisation Agency Guidance in Ear Care. The entire document should be downloaded.[2]

Requirements for ear irrigation

The following items are required:

- chairs for you and the patient

BOX 25.1	Guidance for ear irrigation procedure
1.	Informed consent should be obtained prior to proceeding.
2.	Examine both ears by first inspecting the pinna, outer meatus (ear canal) and adjacent scalp by direct light. Check for previous surgery incision scars or skin defects, then inspect the external ear with the auriscope.
3.	Check whether the patient has had his or her ears irrigated previously and if there are any contraindications (Box 25.2).
4.	Explain the procedure and ask the patient to sit in an examination chair with their head tilted towards the affected ear – a child could sit on an adult's knee with the child's head held steady.
5.	Place the protective cape and towel on the patient's shoulder and under the ear to be irrigated. Ask the patient to hold the receiver under the same ear.
6.	Check that your headlight is in place and the light is directed down the ear canal. Check that the temperature of the water is approximately 40°C and fill the reservoir of the irrigator. Set the pressure at minimum.
7.	Connect clean jet tip applicator to tubing of machine with firm push/twist action. Push until the click is felt.
8.	Direct the irrigator tip into the Noots receiver and switch on the machine for 10–20 seconds in order to circulate the water through the system and eliminate any trapped air or cold water. This offers the opportunity for the patient to become accustomed to the noise of the machine and for you to check the temperature of the water is at 37°C. The initial flow of water is discarded, thus removing any static water remaining in the tube. Every time the irrigator tip is placed in the machine holder water will run back to the canister and the line will have to be reprimed prior to use.
9.	Twist the jet tip so that the water can be aimed along the posterior wall of the ear canal – towards the back of the patient's head.
10.	Gently pull the pinna upwards and outwards to straighten the ear canal – directly backwards in children.
11.	Warn the patient that you are about to start irrigating and that the procedure will be stopped if they feel dizzy or have any pain. Figure 25.1 shows the position of the irrigator. Place the tip of the nozzle into the ear canal entrance and, using foot control, direct the stream of water along the roof of the ear canal and towards the posterior canal wall (directed towards the back of the patient's head). If you consider the entrance to the ear canal as a clock face you would direct the water at 11 o'clock on the right ear and 1 o'clock on the left ear. Increase the pressure control gradually if there is difficulty removing the wax. It is advisable that a maximum of two reservoirs of water are used in any one irrigating procedure.
12.	If you have not managed to remove the wax within 5 minutes of irrigating, it may be worthwhile moving onto the other ear as the introduction of water via the irrigating procedure will soften the wax and you can retry irrigation after about 15 minutes.
13.	Periodically inspect the ear canal with the otoscope and inspect the solution running into the receiver.

Continued

BOX 25.1 *Continued*
14. After removal of wax or debris, dry mop excess water from the meatus under direct vision using the Jobson Horne probe and best quality cotton wool (see Chapter 24). Stagnation of water and any abrasion of skin during the procedure predispose to infection. Removing the water with the cotton-wool-tipped probe reduces the risk of infection.
15. Examine the ear, both meatus and tympanic membrane, and treat as required following specific guidelines, or refer to doctor if necessary.
16. Give advice regarding ear care and any relevant information.
17. Document what was seen in both ears, the procedure carried out, the condition of the tympanic membrane and external auditory meatus, and treatment given. Findings should be recorded according to the NMC guidelines on record keeping and accountability. If any abnormality is found a referral should be made to the ENT outpatient department following local policy.

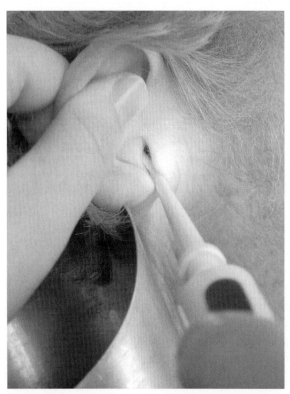

Figure 25.1 The position of the irrigator tip in the ear canal.

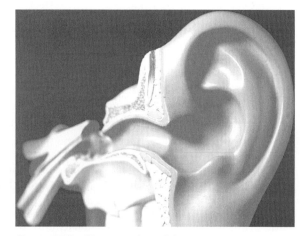

Figure 25.2 Cross-section of the ear.

- otoscope
- head mirror and light or headlight and spare batteries
- electronic irrigator
- jug containing tap water to 40°C
- Noots trough/receiver – a kidney dish does not collect the water and debris sufficiently
- Jobson Horne probe and cotton wool
- tissues and receivers for dirty swabs and instruments
- waterproof cape and towel – I often use a disposable apron placed around the patient's shoulders and tucked into the collar with tissue.

Irrigation should never cause pain. If the patient complains of pain stop immediately.

The parent or guardian should be able to hold the child steady as for immunizations, they should have a full understanding of the procedure and, of course, consent must be given. Educate the parents or guardians not to use anything to clean the child's ear canal. If there is wax in the bowl outside the ear canal (concha) it can be gently wiped with a dry tissue or baby wipe.

BOX 25.2   Contraindications to irrigation

- The patient has previously experienced complications following this procedure in the past
- There is a history of a middle ear infection in the last 6 weeks
- The patient has undergone *any* form of ear surgery (apart from grommets that have extruded at least 18 months previously and the patient has been discharged from the ENT department)
- The patient has a perforation or there is a history of a mucous discharge in the last year
- The patient has a cleft palate (repaired or not)
- The presence of acute otitis externa with pain and tenderness of the pinna
- The patient will not sit still with a steady head for the ear examination

---

EAR IRRIGATION IN CHILDREN

Ear irrigation in children has been described as a vicious cycle, as it may result in repeat procedures being needed. Ear wax and debris are migrated quickly out of the ear canal in children and problems are less common. Accumulation often occurs as a result of parents using cotton buds.

Use your clinical judgement on the most appropriate method to soften the wax. Olive oil should help the wax migrate naturally out of the canal (see Chapter 24). A potential treatment for a young or uncooperative child is for the parents to instil two drops of olive oil into the child's ear at night, when they are asleep on their side. Alternate the ear the following night, and continue for one week.

Irrigation should be a last resort as the child needs to sit still for an ear examination, followed by approximately 10 minutes of irrigation and then a repeat ear examination. There are not many children under the age of five who would stay still for that period of time; however, an individual assessment should be made regardless of age.

POST-IRRIGATION ADVICE

Patients feel that wax is dirty. This way of thinking needs to be changed. It is vital to have some wax in the ear canal to protect and lubricate it. Removal is necessary only if:

- it is causing discomfort
- to aid visibility of the drum, prior to an audiological assessment
- there is potential for an infection to be triggered behind the wax.

ESSENTIAL SKILLS

- An understanding of the anatomy and physiology of the ear and ability to apply this to patient education
- The ability to carry out an ear examination using an otoscope
- The ability to recognize a normal tympanic membrane
- The ability to assess wax/debris in the ear canal and understand the options for removal
- The ability to assess appropriateness of ear irrigation or aural toilet for each patient
- The ability to carry out ear irrigation using appropriate equipment and technique
- The ability to advise patients on post-irrigation care
- Familiarity with the referral process for patients with problems related to the ear and/or hearing

I explain to the patient that removing all the wax from the ear canal by irrigation can make the ear vulnerable until the wax-producing glands secrete enough wax to return the ear canal to its naturally protected state.

It is therefore advisable to keep the ear dry for 4 or 5 days by avoiding washing hair, swimming, showering and bathing, and by placing cotton wool coated in petroleum jelly or ear plugs into the outside of the ear canal. I have found this reduces otitis externa or irritation from shampoos and soaps and helps the patient to understand the importance of wax.

REFERENCES

1. Price J. Problems of ear syringing. Practice Nurse 1997; 14(2): 126–127.
2. Action on ENT Steering Board. Ear Care Guidance Document. London: NHS. Available at: http://www.entnursing.com; http://www.earcarecentre.com; http://www.modern.nhs.uk.

FURTHER READING

Harkin H. Evidence based ear care. Primary Health Care 2000; 10(8): 25–30.

Harkin H. Ear care guide unveiled. Primary Health Care 2002; 12(9): 20.

Harkin H, Vaz FM. The provision of ear care by the practice nurse in the primary health care setting. Primary Health Care 2000; 10(10): 30–33.

Rodgers R. Understanding the legalities of ear syringing. Practice Nurse 2000; 19(4): 166–169.

Chapter 26

An overview of wound management

Maureen Benbow

Wound management has advanced from gauze and mercurochrome to silver and vacuum assisted wound closure (VAC therapy) in a relatively short period of time. Wound management is now a complex and sophisticated area of clinical practice. The number of patients with chronic wounds is increasing in line with the ageing population. This change requires clinicians to spend more time assessing and evaluating the effects of novel treatments and questioning the efficacy of traditional wound-management methods. This is a fascinating time for those with an interest in wound management, as varied therapy options become available. However, there are still misconceptions about appropriate use of wound-management products, and the incorporation of new ideas has been slow.[1, 2]

Nurses and doctors still have much to learn about the principles of moist wound healing, such as:

- product choice
- availability
- composition
- mode of action
- indications and contraindications
- product wear time
- expected outcomes.[3]

They are faced with claims by product manufacturers about rate of wound healing, cost-effectiveness and convenience. What we must remember is that products and devices do not heal wounds. We must ensure that the patient is in the best condition for healing to occur, and correct environmental factors that militate against healing. Justification for the use of the newer therapies is sometimes difficult, as there is little in the way of a sound evidence base to support company claims, and what there is must be challenged. Selecting the most appropriate wound-management product takes knowledge and skill. This chapter focuses on the manage-ment of a range of mostly chronic wounds with a variety of therapies.

WOUNDS

A wound is a break in the epidermis or dermis that can be related to trauma or to pathological changes within the skin or body.[4] It can be acute or chronic. Examples of acute wounds include lacerations, surgical wounds and burns, which usually heal through an orderly sequence of physiological events in a timely fashion, given the appropriate conditions for healing. A chronic wound is any wound that has remained unhealed for more than 6 weeks, usually because of complex underlying pathology such as:

- unrelieved pressure
- malnutrition
- inadequate vascular supply
- diabetes.[4]

Examples are pressure ulcers, leg ulcers and diabetic foot ulcers.

Wounds can be further classified by depth and clinical appearance, which will guide the choice of clinical management. *Full thickness* would be damage penetrating the epidermis, dermis, subcutaneous tissue, fascia and muscle, for example in a cavity wound. *Partial thickness* describes damage penetrating the epidermis and into the dermis, for example a blister or abrasion. *Burns* may be described by the extent of the body burned and the depth of the burn injury. Pressure ulcers and diabetic foot ulcers have their own staging and classification systems.[5, 6]

ASSESSING THE PATIENT

Comprehensive wound assessment is essential to identify both the cause and the factors that may militate against healing. Wound care may be well organized, evidence based and appropriate but, if

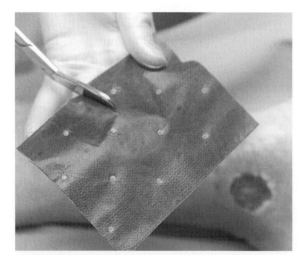

Figure 26.1 Cutting the dressing to size.

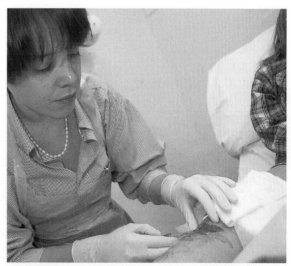

Figure 26.2 Irrigation of a wound.

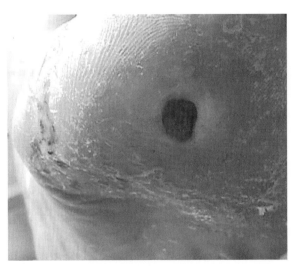

Figure 26.3   Pressure ulcer on a foot.

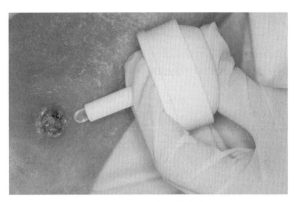

Figure 26.4   Hydrogel being instilled into a wound.

wound aetiology, location, size, exudate and tissue type should be recorded.[10]

the underlying cause is not dealt with, all efforts towards healing are doomed to fail. A useful model to assess the wound and the patient is the 'nine Cs' (Box 26.1).[7]

Wound assessment must include ongoing observation, questioning, data collection and documentation. A wound assessment chart is the best way to achieve consistent documentation. [8, 9] As a minimum, information about the patient,

CHOOSING THE RIGHT DRESSING

Dressings and therapy choice should be based on the findings from the wound assessment. However, dressings can only facilitate wound healing by providing the optimal local environment for healing to proceed – there is no dressing available that can compensate for an uncorrected

BOX 26.1   The nine Cs of wound assessment
1. Cause of the wound (e.g. trauma, pressure, venous insufficiency, malignancy)
2. Clear picture of what the wound looks like (e.g. sloughy, necrotic, granulating, epithelializing, infected)
3. Comprehensive picture of the patient (e.g. medical history, home circumstances and family support, functional capabilities, medication, other treatments such as radiotherapy, physical assessment to identify old scars, ulcers and previous surgery)
4. Contributing factors (e.g. diabetes mellitus, cardiovascular disease, peripheral vascular disease, anaemia)
5. Communication to other healthcare professionals to agree realistic goals
6. Continuity of care – ensuring information passes between healthcare professionals and carers
7. Centralized location for wound care information (e.g. easily accessed, up-to-date, wound care folder, internet and intranet resources)
8. Components of the wound care plan
9. Complications from the wound[7]

pathological condition. Tissue repair will only occur in the presence of adequate oxygen and nutrients, and in the absence of factors that hinder healing. The latter include:

- impaired cardiovascular and pulmonary function
- impaired nutrition and fluid intake
- metabolic conditions
- diabetes
- steroids
- smoking
- immunosuppression
- advancing age.[9, 11–15]

Moist wound healing

George Winter pioneered the development of modern wound management products. Using an animal model he demonstrated that epidermal repair was twice as fast for wounds covered with a vapour-permeable film dressing compared with those left to scab over.[3] In later studies the natural process of autolysis (the breaking down of devitalized tissue) was enhanced in a moist environment and local wound pain control was also achieved.[16–18]

Many modern wound-management products provide the moist, clean and warm environment for healing. Moisture, however, can cause maceration of the surrounding skin. It is often the fine balance between wet and dry at the wound surface that is difficult to achieve.

Dressing requirements

Wound dressing has become a very complex, sophisticated and expensive issue. The unit cost of modern wound management products is high, compared with traditional dressings. However, this must be weighed against cost-effectiveness of fast healing and improving the patient's quality of life.[19] Many of the modern wound-management products require infrequent changes and, there-

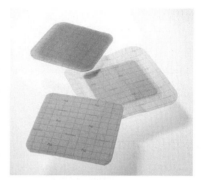

Figure 26.5 Selection of dressings.

fore, interfere less with the patient's lifestyle and wound healing.

Nurses require dressings that:

- maintain high humidity at the wound/dressing interface
- remove excess exudate
- allow gaseous exchange
- provide thermal insulation
- are impermeable to bacteria
- are free of particles and toxic wound contaminants
- allow removal without causing trauma to the wound.[20]

Several more criteria could be added, for example to prevent damage to the surrounding skin, to be acceptable to the patient and to be inexpensive for budget-holders. Issues such as ease of application and removal, conformability and comfort can make a big difference to patient concordance.

> ### ESSENTIAL SKILLS
>
> - Know how to assess the patient and the wound
> - Understand the principles of wound care
> - Knowledge of the factors that hinder healing
> - Understand the principles of moist wound healing
> - Know the requirements of a dressing
> - Knowledge of the local wound dressing formulary

CONCLUSION

Dressing choice should be based on wound assessment and on the principles of wound care.[7] Practice nurses need to keep themselves updated about the latest products and advances in tissue viability. Local evidence-based treatment protocols and guidelines need to be available to help ensure best practice.

REFERENCES

1. Benbow M. Mixing and matching dressing products. Nursing Standard 2000; 14(49): 56–62.
2. Benbow M. Mixing dressings – a clinical governance issue? J Commun Nursing 2004; 18(3): 27–32.
3. Winter GD. Formation of the scab and the rate of epithelialisation of superficial wounds in the skin of the domestic pig. Nature 1962; 193: 293.
4. Collins F, Hampton S, White R. A–Z Dictionary of Wound Care. London: Quay Books, 2000.
5. European Pressure Ulcer Advisory Panel. Pressure Ulcer Treatment Guidelines. Oxford: EPUAP, 1999.
6. Wagner FW Jr. The dysvascular foot: a system for diagnosis and treatment. Foot Ankle 1981; 2(2): 64–122.
7. Baranowski S, Ayello EA. Wound Care Essentials. Practice Principles. London: Lippincott, 2004.
8. Banfield KR, Shuttleworth E. A systematic approach with lasting benefits: designing a wound assessment chart. Professional Nurse 1993; 8(4): 234–238.
9. Morison M. A Colour Guide to the Nursing Management of Wounds. London: Wolfe, 1992.
10. Flanagan M. Improving the accuracy of wound measurement in clinical practice. Ostomy Wound Manage 2003: 49(10): 28–40.
11. Bryant R (ed.). Acute and Chronic Wounds. Nursing Management. London: Mosby Year Book, 2000.
12. Cutting K. Factors influencing healing. Nursing Standard 1994; 8(50): 33–36.
13. Flanagan M. Wound Care Society Educational Leaflet. No. 5. Huntingdon: Wound Care Society, 1989.
14. Dealey C. The Care of Wounds. A Guide for Nurses, 2nd edn. Oxford: Blackwell Science, 2000.
15. Doughty B. Principles of wound healing and wound management. In: Bryant R. Acute and Chronic Wounds. Nursing Management. London: Mosby Year Book, 2000.
16. Friedman S, Su DWP. Hydrocolloid occlusive dressing management of leg ulcers. Arch Dermatol 1982; 120(3): 1329–1331.
17. Alvarez O, Rozint J, Wiseman D. Moist environment for healing: matching the dressing to the wound. Wounds 1989; 1(1): 35–51.
18. Eaglstein WH. Experiences with biosynthetic dressings. J Am Acad Dermatol 1985; 12(2 Pt 2); 434–440.
19. Hampton S. Choosing the right dressing. In: Miller M, Glover D (eds). Wound Management: Theory and Practice. London: NT Books; 1999, pp 116–128.
20. Turner TD. Which dressing and why? Nursing Times 1982; 78(29 Suppl): 1–3.

Chapter 27

Wound management materials

Maureen Benbow

Dressing choice should be based on wound assessment and on the principles of wound care (see Chapter 26). There are a range of wound management materials available.

LOW-ADHERENT DRESSINGS

Dressings such as Melolin, Release and NA Ultra can be regarded as low-adherent (rather than non-adherent) dressings. Most nurses will have had experience of their sticking to open wounds. They should only be used for wounds with low levels of exudate, or be used as carriers for hydrogels on sloughy or necrotic wounds covered with a semi-permeable film dressing. NA Ultra is recommended when adherence to the wound is a potential problem.[1]

Medicated low-adherent dressings – such as Inadine, which is impregnated with povidone–iodine – are indicated for shallow, open, clinically infected wounds. This would include minor burns, superficial skin loss injuries and diabetic ulcers. Inadine should be avoided in patients with sensitivity to iodine or povidone–iodine.

Exudate levels dictate the frequency of dressing changes. If a large volume of exudate is being produced, daily changing will probably be needed. Therapeutic antibacterial levels are unlikely after 2 days.[1]

In my experience, adherence can be a problem, in which case the dressing can be loosened with warmed saline.

OPTIMIZING HEALING

The main groups of modern products that provide the optimum wound-healing environment are semipermeable film dressings, hydrogels, hydro-colloids, alginates, foams and hydrofibre dressings. If chosen appropriately, dressings from each group will assist healing and debridement.

Film dressings

Film dressings, such as Tegaderm, Op-site and C-View, usually consist of a thin polyurethane membrane coated with a layer of acrylic adhesive (usually hypoallergenic).[1]

They are permeable to water vapour and oxygen but impermeable to bacteria, ensuring that the wound-healing environment remains clean, warm and moist. Moisture prevents the development of a scab on the wound surface, and the pain caused by the exposure of nerve endings is reduced within this environment.

Films are useful as secondary dressings to cover hydrogels, alginates and hydrofibre dressings to prevent them drying out. It is possible to observe the wound through these transparent dressings without removal. Many film products have novel designs to aid their application. Films have limited absorbency, and should therefore only be used as primary dressings for non-clinically infected, shallow, low-exudate wounds, such as pressure ulcers, minor burns, lacerations and abrasions. I also find these products useful to reduce friction and to protect vulnerable skin.

Application

Manufacturer's recommendations for application, removal and wear time of film dressings should be followed. They should not be stretched or the skin will wrinkle after application. There are also special techniques to apply films to awkward places, such as the heel or elbow, by cutting and applying the film in strips, or shaping it to fit around fingers and hands comfortably. Film dressings can be left in place for up to 7 days, depending on the level of exudate and how well they adhere.

Removal

When removing a film dressing, an edge should be lifted and the body of the dressing stretched parallel to the skin in the direction of hair growth (Figure 27.1). The rest of the dressing should be supported with the other hand. In between each stretch, relax the film and then stretch it again to break down the adhesive. This will prevent trauma to the surrounding skin and wound.

Amorphous hydrogels

Amorphous hydrogels such as Intrasite, Nu-gel and Granugel mainly consist of water (approximately 80–94%), with polymer, humectant and preservative. They donate fluid to rehydrate dead tissue when placed in contact with a wound. The main indications are for sloughy, dry, necrotic wounds, such as pressure ulcers, leg ulcers, extravasation injuries and surgical wounds. Hydrogels can, however, be used effectively throughout healing on low-exudate granulating and epithe-lializing wounds.

They do not absorb fluid and, therefore, are not recommended for wet wounds. A secondary dressing is always needed. Ideally, they should be

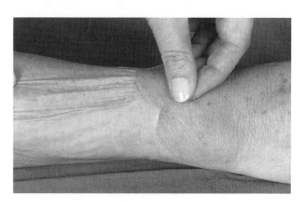

Figure 27.1   Removal of a film dressing.

covered with a semipermeable film dressing to prevent the gel drying out and to aid autolytic debridement. The frequency of dressing changes will depend on the state of the wound and effectiveness of desloughing. On drier wounds, hydrogels may be left for up to 3 days.[1] Again, there are different presentations available, such as Intrasite Conformable.

Hydrocolloids

Hydrocolloids, such as Duoderm, Cutinova Hydro and Comfeel Plus, are interactive dressings. They generally consist of cellulose, gelatine and pectin, with a polyurethane film or foam backing. They are self-adhesive and are indicated for wounds with low to medium levels of exudate, such as pressure ulcers, leg ulcers, minor burns and traumatic wounds.

Properties

They can absorb and hold moderate amounts of exudate in the hydrocolloid matrix. Hydrocolloids are impermeable to water vapour, allowing the patient to bath or shower with the dressing in place. They help in rehydration and autolytic debridement of necrotic and sloughy wounds.

Application and removal

Wound pain is reduced when the dressing is in place, and removal is usually atraumatic if the dressing is removed by pulling back on itself, like removing a sticking plaster. Application and adhesion is facilitated by warming the dressing between your hands prior to application and when in place. The hypoxic environment created by hydrocolloids is said to encourage angiogenesis.[2]

A common problem with adhesive dressings is rolling of the edges, particularly when applied to the sacrum if the patient moves about. This can be prevented by careful application and a small amount of talcum powder applied to the sticky edges. A general rule is that hydrocolloids should not be left in place for more than 7 days.[1]

Product range

Hydrocolloids are available in many different presentations for both flat wounds and cavity wounds. A newer adaptation is Aquacel, which is a highly absorbent flat-sheet dressing or ribbon made of hydrocolloid fibres. It forms a thick conformable gel when it absorbs exudate.[3] Cutinova Cavity and Aquacel are both suitable for heavily to moderately exuding wounds.[4] Urgotul is another useful hydrocolloid variation (lipidocolloid). It is non-adherent and can be left for up to 14 days as a wound contact layer.[5]

Alginates

Alginates. such as Kaltostat, Sorbsan and SeaSorb, are derived from different types of seaweed, and are suitable for moderately to heavily exuding wounds. The fibrous dressing forms a gel when it absorbs exudate, to provide a suitable environment for healing.

Kaltostat is also licensed as a haemostat, most usefully for exuding cavity wounds. Alginates need a secondary dressing to contain moisture and aid autolysis.

These dressings are easily removed in one piece – with a gloved finger or forceps – or irrigated out of the wound. Dressing change intervals will be dependent upon the exudate levels, but alginates should not be left in place for longer than 7 days on a non-infected wound.[1]

Polyurethane foam dressings

Polyurethane foam dressings, such as Allevyn and Tielle, are made of polyurethane or silicone, and are used as flat dressings or as fillers for cavity wounds (Figure 27.2). They can be adhesive or non-adhesive.

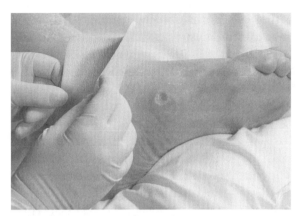

Figure 27.2   Application of a foam dressing.

The interface with the wound is constructed so that it takes up large amounts of blood and exudate by capillary action into or across the dressing. Some foam dressings have an outer vapour-permeable polyurethane film backing. They are indicated for moderately to heavily exuding wounds, and adherent foam dressings provide an effective barrier to bacteria. The construction of the contact layer of the dressing ensures that it will not stick to the surface of the wound.

Non-adherent foams should be held in place with thin strips of adhesive tape along the edges, or with a retaining bandage. On a clean, non-infected wound, the dressings can be left in place for 4–5 days.[1]

Foams will not provide any therapeutic benefit for dry necrotic wounds. Foam sheet dressings are frequently used as secondary dressings over alginates and hydrofibre dressings, when extra absorbency is required. There are various shapes and sizes available that attempt to meet the demands of all types and locations of wounds.

Cavi-care

Cavi-care (formerly Silastic foam) is a foam product. It must be mixed with a catalyst before being poured into a wound cavity where it takes on the shape of the wound.

Other dressings

Charcoal dressings

Charcoal dressings, such as Actisorb Silver 2000, Carboflex, Carbonet and Lyofoam Care, are constructed of activated charcoal cloth, and work by absorbing the chemicals released from malodorous wounds.

The inclusion of silver in Actisorb Silver 2000 is said to attract bacteria into the dressing away from the wound. Several new silver-containing dressings are now available for infected wounds, in the form of foams (Contreet), hydrocolloid (Contreet), hydrofibre (Aquacel Ag) or wound contact layers (Acticoat, Urgotul Sag).

Antibacterials include Flamazine and Metrotop gel. Flamazine, a cream containing 1% silver sulphadiazine, is effective against a wide range of bacteria, and is commonly used for burns and leg ulceration.

Metrotop gel contains metronidazole (0.8%), and is an effective deodorizer for pressure ulcers, fungating wounds and other lesions infected with anaerobic organisms. For clinically infected wounds, appropriate antibiotic cover is necessary. Metrotop gel is normally used in conjunction with systemic metronidazole for best effect.

Skin protectants

Maceration and damage to the surrounding skin is a major problem associated with chronic and infected wounds and their frequent redressing.

Cavilon has, over the last few years, become a popular and effective addition to many formularies for protecting skin prior to the application of adhesive dressings. It is also useful in the treatment of excoriated, macerated skin due to incontinence, oral dribbling and leaking stomas.

Cavilon barrier film, supplied as either a spray or swab, should be applied to the affected skin and left to dry for 30 seconds. One application should last for 2–3 days, depending on the level of moisture present and frequency of cleansing.

Cavilon cream is also available for prophylaxis in patients with at-risk skin.

Tulle dressings are less popular than they used to be. When they are used as primary dressings, granulation tissue grows into the open weave of the tulle and is torn away when the dressing is removed. They also dry out quickly. These products have largely been superseded by modern wound-management products.

WOUND INFECTION AND DRESSINGS

Infected wounds must be treated symptomatically. The main problems will usually be excess exudate and odour. If clinical infection is suspected, it should be confirmed microbiologi-cally and systemic antibiotics prescribed.

Modern wound-management products can be used in conjunction with antibiotics, but high exudate levels in infected wounds will dictate frequent dressing changes. It is advisable to check an infected wound daily while exudate levels are high and malodour is a problem.

Certain dressings, such as Duoderm, Granuflex, Tegaderm and Tegasorb, are not recommended for use on clinically infected wounds (see Surgical Materials Testing Laboratory (SMTL) Data Cards at http://www.smtl.co.uk).

If you are in doubt about using a particular dressing on a clinically infected wound, contact the company helpline or local representative. As the infection resolves, exudate will decrease, and dressings may then be left in place for longer periods.

Dressings containing silver are proving to be effective in managing infected wounds.

ACCOUNTABILITY, TRAINING AND PROFESSIONAL INDEMNITY

The NMC Code of Professional Conduct (2002) states that as a registered nurse, midwife or health visitor you are personally accountable for your practice. You must:

- obtain consent before you give any treatment or care
- maintain your professional knowledge and competence
- act to identify and minimize risk to patients and clients.

The patient needs to have the options explained to them, and must be in full agreement with any wound treatment. A patient may choose to refuse a treatment, such as larval therapy (where maggots are applied to a wound), without jeopardizing their future care.

Patients must also give oral consent, or in some cases written consent (according to local protocols), to their wound being photographed. They must also be told what the photographs will be used for (e.g. teaching, or as illustrations in case studies).

Nurses must never apply a treatment for which they have not been trained. You need to know how the treatment works and the consequences of its use, as well as how to apply and remove it safely.

Making sure you are up-to-date in your knowledge of tissue viability is essential to ensure correct and safe treatment and successful outcomes. Local evidence-based treatment protocols and guidelines should be readily available to ensure best practice.

CONCLUSION

The range of wound-care products increases daily and, with the advent of more advanced technologies, it can be a challenge to justify and defend the choices made. Decisions will be needed about whether technologies such as vacuum-assisted therapy, hyperbaric oxygen, larval therapy, or even alternative and complementary therapies, become part of nursing wound management. In the meantime, nurses must familiarize themselves with commonly used treatments to ensure that wound management follows best practice.

ESSENTIAL SKILLS

- Knowledge of the range of dressings available and their indications
- Ability to correctly apply and remove each type of dressing
- Understanding of informed consent and how to ensure it is obtained

---

REFERENCES

1. Thomas S. Handbook of Wound Dressings. London: Macmillan Magazines, 1994.
2. Cherry GW, Ryan TJ. Enhanced wound angiogenesis with a new hydrocolloid dressing. Royal Society of Medicine International Congress and Symposium Series 1985; 88: 5–14.
3. Flanagan M. Wound Management. Edinburgh: Churchill Livingstone, 1997.
4. Dealey C. The Care of Wounds. A Guide for Nurses, 2nd edn. Oxford: Blackwell Science, 2000.
5. Benbow M, Iosson G. A clinical evaluation of the use of Urgotul in the treatment of acute and chronic wounds. Br J Nurs 2004;13(2): 105–109.

Chapter 28

Doppler readings and leg ulceration

Maureen Benbow

It was an Austrian mathematician living in the 19th century who defined the Doppler principle. J. Christian Doppler's theory states that an apparent shift in transmitted frequency occurs as a result of motion of either the source or the target. One example of this is the increase in frequency of sound produced by a motorbike travelling towards you, and then the decrease in frequency as it moves away. Today, the Doppler principle forms the basis of one of the most important assessment parameters used to aid the diagnosis of leg ulceration (Figure 28.1).

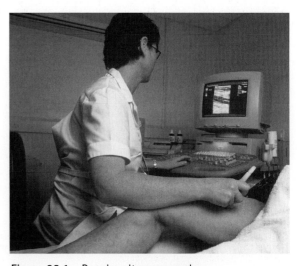

Figure 28.1   Doppler ultrasonography.

LEG ULCERS

Leg ulcers are an increasingly common chronic wound.[1] The successful management of leg ulcers has developed over recent years to the point where early identification of the underlying aetiology and appropriate treatment will heal many, formerly recalcitrant, ulcers.

Leg ulceration in women in later life is often connected with deep vein damage due to thrombosis during pregnancy, which may explain why more women than men develop ulcers.[2] Leg ulceration affects between 1% and 2% of the UK population. This equates to 80,000–100,000 people suffering from an open wound at a given time and 400,000 people with a healed ulcer that is likely to recur.[3, 4]

AETIOLOGY OF LEG ULCERS

The origin of approximately 70% of all ulcers is predominantly chronic venous insufficiency caused by incompetent valves in the deep and

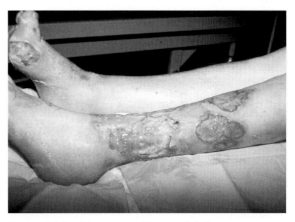

Figure 28.2   Ulcers caused by arterial disease are most common on the foot.

perforating veins.[4] The second most common cause of leg ulceration is arteriosclerotic occlusion of the large vessels of the legs (arterial ulcers) leading to ischaemia, with a third group comprising damage caused by chronic venous hypertension and arterial disease (mixed ulcers). Table 28.1 shows the different clinical presentations of ulceration of venous and arterial aetiology (Figure 28.2).

TABLE 28.1   Clinical presentation of ulceration due to venous and arterial disease

	Arterial disease	Venous disease
Site	Anywhere, but more common on the foot	Most frequently around the medial malleolus
Pain	Increased at night, with exercise or when the legs are elevated	Dull, aching, relieved by elevation
Skin colour	Legs pale and hairless	Characteristic brown staining above medial malleolus
Oedema	Often seen when legs are dependent	Worse in the evening, reduces with elevation
Toes	Poor capillary refill/cyanosed	–
Veins	–	Often distended
Ulcer	Punched out, deep, with extensive tissue loss	Shallow and flat, high exudate
Eczema	–	Can be wet, dry, localized or general
Pulses	ABPI < 0.8	ABPI > 0.9
History	Smoking, etc.	Deep vein thrombosis, phlebitis, varicose veins, surgery

ABPI, ankle brachial pressure index

Leg ulceration may also be associated with a variety of other disease entities:

- neuropathy associated with diabetes
- vasculitis associated with rheumatoid arthritis
- malignancy (squamous cell carcinoma, melanoma)
- blood disorders (polycythaemia, sickle-cell disease)
- infection (tuberculosis)
- metabolic disorders (pyoderma gangrenosum)
- lymphoedema
- trauma
- iatrogenic (tight bandaging)
- self-inflicted.[2]

ASSESSMENT OF THE PATIENT WITH LOWER LIMB ULCERATION

A comprehensive medical history should be taken prior to local assessment, to include identification of any significant indicators for venous or arterial disease. Stroke, transient ischaemic attacks, angina or myocardial infarction may predispose to arterial impairment, and intermittent claudication is invariably associated with poor perfusion in the lower limbs.[5]

Level of mobility, nutritional status, sleep position, smoking and pain are just some of the risk factors that should be explored with the patient. Also establish the patient's attitude to the ulcer.

You should test urine to rule out diabetes and check the haemoglobin level to rule out anaemia. Examination of the legs may reveal classic signs of chronic venous insufficiency such as lipodermatosclerosis in the gaiter area and/or ankle flare. There may be gangrene of the toes, with cold, hairless skin.

Palpation of the foot pulses is not a reliable method for testing the arterial status of a patient.[6] It should not be relied upon alone because:

- there will be variance between assessors

- the pedal pulses may be bounding in a diabetic patient with arterial compromise nearer the toes
- there may be congenital absence of the dorsalis pedis in 12% of people[7]
- the presence of oedema will make palpation difficult.[6]

A more reliable tentative differential diagnosis can be made between venous and arterial ulceration by assessment of the blood supply to the leg using Doppler ultrasonography to calculate the ankle brachial pressure index (ABPI).

ABPI

Training and assessment of competence is required before a clinician carries out the procedure of calculating the ankle brachial pressure index (Box 28.1). The ABPI measurement is an essential component of vascular assessment of the leg combined with a detailed and accurate physical examination.

Clinical examination and palpation of pedal pulses are insufficient to support an accurate diagnosis and the danger is that compression therapy may be initiated inappropriately.[2, 5, 8, 9]

The ABPI ratio is used to exclude the likelihood of significant peripheral arterial disease. However, the ABPI is not indicative of microvascular disease, vasculitis or diabetes, and can give rise to misleading falsely high ratios in diabetic patients.

Method

Assessment of the ABPI is carried out using a hand-held Doppler ultrasound and should be carried out on all patients presenting with lower limb ulceration. This is to assess the adequacy of the peripheral circulation and whether any significant arterial disease is present prior to establishing a treatment plan. The recommended probes are 8 MHz for normal-sized limbs and 5 MHz for obese or oedematous limbs.[10]

BOX 28.1   The technique of ABPI measurement

1. • Explain the procedure and reassure the patient.

2. • Allow the patient to lie comfortably and as flat as possible with no pressure on the limbs.

3. • Allow the patient to rest for 10–20 minutes to ensure the systolic pressure is not artificially raised due to exertion.

4. • Place a sphygmomanometer cuff around the upper arm and locate the brachial pulse by palpation and apply ultrasound gel (not KY jelly).
   • Angle the transducer (probe) at 45° and locate the best signal.
   • Inflate the cuff until the signal disappears.
   • Deflate slowly and record the pressure at which the signal returns.
   • Repeat for the other arm and use the higher value to calculate the ABPI.

5. • Place the (appropriately sized) cuff around the leg immediately above the ankle, covering any ulceration with a dressing or thin film.
   • Locate the dorsalis pedis, apply gel and continue as above.
   • Repeat for the posterior tibial pulse.

6. • Use the higher reading to calculate the ABPI for that leg, repeat the measurement on the other leg

7. • The pressure in the leg is divided by the systolic pressure in the arm to produce the ABPI:

   $$ABPI = \frac{\text{Higher of the 2 ankle pressures}}{\text{Higher of the 2 brachial pressures}}$$

8. • A pressure index of < 0.8 is suggestive of arterial disease; an ABPI of 0.4–0.5 denotes severe arterial disease; ABPI below 0.4 (only 40% of the possible blood flow is managing to get through the artery) denotes critical ischaemia and is a surgical emergency.

9. • The degenerative arterial effects of diabetes or oedema can skew the accuracy of the reading.

   Example:
   Ankle = 100
   Brachial = 140
   ABPI = 100/140 = 0.71

   Arteries have a strong pulsating sound that is usually triphasic but often only two phases (biphasic) might be heard, while veins do not pulsate but give a 'whooshing' or roaring sound.

Safety or accuracy will not be compromised in the presence of ulceration or oedema in the ankle region during Doppler assessment if the ulceration is appropriately covered. Suitable ultrasound gel should be used to ensure good transmission of the signal and to prevent corrosion of the probe.[11]

The crystal in the probe emits a beam of ultrasound waves that travel to the underlying vessels, where it is reflected by the red blood cells in proportion to the speed of the cells. A second crystal in the probe picks up the returning signal.[11]

Results

In an individual without arterial disease the normal ABPI would be greater than 1.0, which means that there is no obstruction to normal blood flow.

The decision to apply graduated compression bandaging would be made based on this finding plus the findings from the general assessment. However, an ABPI of 0.9–0.95 indicates a degree of arterial disease. Patients found to have a ratio of less than 0.8 should be referred for further vascular assessment. Compression therapy is contraindicated in patients with a ratio of < 0.8.

Abnormally high ratios, i.e. above 1.5, may indicate the presence of medial calcinosis, diabetes, severe oedema and atherosclerosis, and care should be exercised in their management.[11]

The measured ankle cuff pressure may be falsely elevated in diabetic patients with calcified arteries. Peripheral arterial disease may be present if the ABPI is less than 0.95. Many patients with a reduced ABPI are symptom-free. However Table 28.2 gives some idea of the symptoms associated with various severities of peripheral arterial disease.

Summary

- Patients with an ABPI of 0.8 or greater may have compression bandaging or hosiery.
- Patients with an ABPI of 0.6–0.8 have moderate arterial disease. If the ulcer is clinically venous, reduced compression may be used; if the ulcer is clinically non-venous, the causative factors must be considered.
- Patients with an ABPI of less than 0.6 have severe arterial disease and should be referred

immediately for further investigation – compression bandaging must not be applied.[10]

VENOUS ULCERATION

Calculation of the ABPI is conducted to screen for peripheral vascular disease of the legs. However, care should be taken not to use this assessment to diagnose venous ulceration. It may be used as an arbitrary cut-off point to define a safe level of compression bandaging.[12]

As leg venous ulceration commonly occurs in the older age group, it will often coexist with arterial disease over time, hence the need for regular reassessment of the ABPI (every 3 months, or earlier if symptoms change to guide treatment decisions).[10]

In the presence of arterial disease, compression therapy may become inappropriate and lead to local tissue damage. The 0.8 cut-off point for compression therapy does not define the transition between venous and arterial disease or consider pressure differences between the three vessels at the ankle.

Researchers recommend that the ABPI value should not be regarded as an absolute.[13] Other factors should be considered, such as the shape of the limb, correction of the underlying arterial disease and the application of compression, and trying alternative therapies such as pneumatic compression or short stretch bandaging instead of conventional multilayer compression bandaging.[13]

TABLE 28.2 Symptoms associated with various severities of peripheral arterial disease[12]	
Clinical status	**ABPI**
Symptom free	1 or more
Intermittent claudication	0.95–0.5
Rest pain	0.5–0.3
Gangrene and ulceration	0.2

CONCLUSION

Specialist training is required to assess patients with leg ulcers – basic wound management training is not adequate. The competencies needed for undertaking Doppler assessment include a sound in-depth knowledge of the aetiology of leg ulceration, and wound management, assessment, planning, implementation and evaluation skills, and an understanding of what the ulcer means to the patient.

Calculation of the ABPI has been shown to be unreliable when carried out by inexperienced users, which may lead to the application of incorrect treatment.[14]

As nurses are responsible for most of the assessment and management of patients with leg ulcers, constituting a large part of the primary care nurse workload, it is essential that they have the necessary knowledge and skills to do so safely, and to know when to refer on to other healthcare professionals for specialist assessment.

ESSENTIAL SKILLS

- Accurate assessment of the patient
- Specialist Doppler training
- Knowing when to ask for advice from colleagues

REFERENCES

1. Dealey C. The Nursing Care Of Wounds. London: Blackwell Science, 2000.
2. Moffatt C, Franks PJ. A prerequisite underlining the treatment programme. Risk factors associated with venous disease. Professional Nurse 1994; 9(9): 637–640, 642.
3. Laing W. Chronic Venous Diseases of the Leg. London: Office of Health Economics, 1992.
4. Callam MJ, Harper DR, Dale JJ, Ruckley CV. Chronic ulceration of the leg: extent of the problem and provision of care. BMJ 1985: 290(6485);1855–1856.
5. Callam MJ, Harper DR, Dale JJ, Ruckley CV. Chronic ulcer of the leg: clinical history. BMJ 1987: 294(6584); 1389–1391.
6. Morison MJ, Moffatt CJ. A Colour Guide to the Assessment and Management of Leg Ulcers, 2nd edn. London: Mosby, 1994.
7. Barnhorst DA, Barner HB Prevalence of congenitally absent pedal pulses. N Engl J Med 1986; 278(5): 264–265.
8. Bale S, Harding K. Leg ulcers: education for nurses and patients. Nursing Standard 1989; 3(42): 25–27.
9. Cameron J. Dressing leg ulcers. Nurs Elderly 1991; 3(5): 17–19.
10. Royal College of Nursing. Implementation Guide. Clinical Guidelines for the Management of Venous Leg Ulcers. London: RCN, 2000.
11. Morison MJ, Moffatt CJ. Leg ulcers. In: Morison M, Moffatt C, Bridel-Nixon J, Bale S (eds). A Colour Guide to the Nursing Management of Chronic Wounds. London: Mosby, 1997.
12. Gpnotebook. Ankle brachial pressure index. 2003. Available at: http://www.gpnotebook.co.uk/ simplepage.cfm?ID=-1563426745
13. Vowden P, Vowden K. Doppler assessment and ABPI: interpretation in the management of leg ulceration 2001. Available at: http://www.worldwidewounds.com/2001/ march/Vowden/Doppler-assessment
14. Ray SA, Srodon PD, Taylor RS, Dormandy JA. Reliability of ankle brachial pressure index measurement by junior doctors. BMJ 1994; 81(2): 188–190.

Laboratory investigations

Mike McGhee

Performing tests on patients in general practice for infections and haematological and biochemical problems has been part of the service offered by primary healthcare teams for many years. The quantity and variety of tests performed by GPs began to increase about 20 years ago, when the number of practice nurses employed in primary care rose, opening up the possibility of doing more tests in primary care rather than sending patients to hospital. Nowadays many practices employ their own phlebotomists, allowing the practice nurse to carry out other increasingly varied and skilful tasks.

Even in practices that do not perform blood sampling, there is still a need to be able to interpret the results of laboratory tests, which inevitably come back to the patient's GP whether or not that test was requested by the GP in the first instance.

Performing tests in primary care is often very convenient for the patient, and saves time and money for secondary care, but increases the burden on GPs and practice nurses. Primary care trusts (PCTs), however, have recognized the potential cost savings to be made from performing some of these tasks in primary care.

In the new GMS contract, payments can be made to practices for carrying out some tests that were previously almost exclusively undertaken in hospitals, such as blood clotting estimations (international normalized ratio (INR)) in patients taking warfarin. The scope and variety of the treatment of some medical conditions has increased with the ability to carry out more tests in primary care, such as the management of patients with suspected deep vein thrombosis (DVT), who can be managed almost exclusively in primary care when there is the ability to monitor the INR. There is a potential cost saving available to PCTs having this service available in primary care rather than commissioning it from secondary care.

A number of tests that used to be performed only in the hospital laboratory can now be carried out in the GP surgery (near-patient testing), without the need for the sample, or patient, to be transported to hospital. These include urine testing for infection, urinary pregnancy testing and some blood testing, such as haemoglobin estimations, blood glucose, blood cholesterol and INR in patients on warfarin. Cervical cytology has always been mainly carried out in primary care (as well as family planning clinics), but even this process is changing with the introduction of liquid-based cytology.

URINE TESTING

Urine testing used to include only checks for protein and sugar, or blood protein, sugar and ketones, but now includes testing for pH, nitrates, white cells (leucocytes), bilirubin and urobilinogen.

Using Labstix to test the urine for all of the above greatly reduces the number of urine samples that need to be sent to the microbiology laboratory for culture and examination of organisms in cases of suspected infection. For example, a patient with symptoms of dysuria and increased frequency of micturition is unlikely to have a lower urinary tract infection in the absence of leucocytes (white cells), blood or protein. It is therefore probably not necessary to send such a urine sample to hospital for culture and sensitivity of organisms, because it is unlikely that there will be any infection (Figure 29.1 and Box 29.1).

BLOOD TESTS

A very wide variety of blood tests are performed in primary care. The most common blood tests are haematological tests, biochemical tests and immunological tests. Immunological tests such as those used to diagnose coeliac disease are now common in primary care.

In addition there are a number of specialized tests such as tests for fertility and tests performed during pregnancy, virology tests to identify specific infections, and prostate blood testing screening for prostate cancer.

The values given for normal ranges of haematological and biochemical test results vary from laboratory to laboratory, and the reference ranges shown in Boxes 29.2 and 29.3 are given for guidance only. Local values should be observed.

ESSENTIAL SKILLS

- Knowledge of the local protocol for midstream urine samples
- Knowledge of the reference values used by your local laboratory for blood tests

---

FURTHER READING

McGhee M. A Guide to Laboratory Investigations, 4th edn. Oxford: Radcliffe Medical Press, 2003.[Provides a full explanation of all the common laboratory tests.]

BOX 29.1   Urinalysis

- Testing the urine with dipsticks relies upon a chemical reaction occurring between the reagent in the strip and a constituent within the urine
- Dipstick testing is useful for screening patients with possible renal tract (kidney, ureter, bladder and urethra) disease
- Following urine dipstick testing, it may be necessary to send a clean (midstream urine) sample to the laboratory for further diagnosis, especially when identifying an infection

Leucocytes

- Leucocytes are white cells. Their presence in urine may indicate infection
- A trace of leucocytes with negative nitrates, negative or trace protein and negative blood probably indicates contamination and the specimen test should be repeated
- The presence of glucose, albumin and some antibiotics can give a false-negative result

Nitrates

- Most white cells in urine produce a chemical reaction that converts nitrates into nitrites, causing the colour change on the dipstick test
- A positive nitrate test with a positive test for white cells is strongly suggestive of urine infection

Urobilinogen

- Urobilinogen is only of importance in liver disease (see bilirubin)

Protein

- Protein in the urine other than a trace of protein strongly suggests renal disease
- A clean (midstream) urine sample should be sent to the laboratory to detect infection and confirm the presence of protein

pH

- Dipstick testing gives only an approximate estimate of the acidity or alkalinity in the urine. Normal pH varies between 4.5 and 8.0
- Urine pH may be important in patients with kidney stones. Altering the pH may reduce stone formation

Blood

- A very small quantity of blood (red cells) is excreted in the urine but does not normally give a positive dipstick test
- Blood in the urine should always be investigated further with, at least, a clean (midstream) urine test specimen being sent to the laboratory to exclude infection and confirm the presence or absence of red cells
- In women, the most common cause of blood in the urine is menstrual blood loss
- Other causes of blood in the urine are kidney stones, trauma, kidney infection (glomerulonephritis) and cancer

Specific gravity

- Specific gravity indicates the patient's urine concentration and therefore the patient's state of hydration
- Specific gravity testing is not accurate or reliable
- Normal values lie between 1,003 and 1,030
- Specific gravity decreases with age as the kidney loses its concentrating ability

Continued

BOX 29.1   *Continued*

Ketones

- Ketones are present in dehydration and in diabetic ketoacidosis (positive ketones and positive glucose in the urine)
- Ketoacidosis (ketones and glucose both present in the urine) is a life-threatening condition requiring urgent blood sugar measurement and appropriate treatment (insulin)

Bilirubin

- Bilirubin is not normally detectable in the urine except with liver or gallbladder disease
- When the patient is jaundiced (yellow skin due to raised blood bilirubin levels), the presence of bilirubin in the urine suggests liver disease rather than jaundice from other causes

Glucose

- Glucose should not normally be present in the urine and occurs either because the blood sugar level is high (diabetes mellitus) or because glucose leaks from the kidney (renal glycosuria), which can occur in healthy kidneys (e.g. during pregnancy) or in diseased kidneys
- When glucose is detected in the urine (glycosuria), a fasting blood sugar test should always be performed

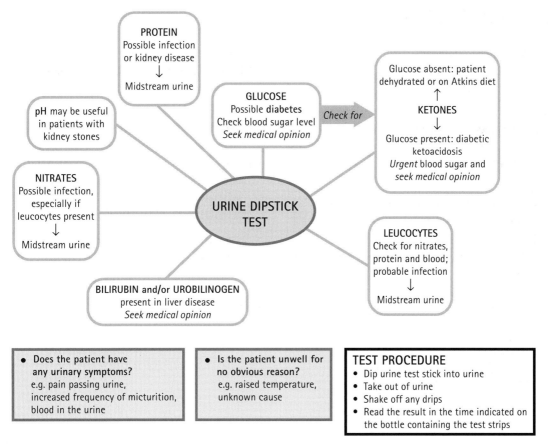

Figure 29.1   Urine dipstick testing.

BOX 29.2   Haematological tests

Haemoglobin

- Haemoglobin measurement is the test for anaemia (low haemoglobin) or polycythaemia (high haemoglobin). The level of haemoglobin in an individual remains fairly constant, but can vary significantly between two individuals. The level in children varies with age, sex and race

- Anaemia is the cause of a low haemoglobin level, and further tests are usually performed, such as serum iron, vitamin B_{12} and folate, to help determine the cause of the anaemia and instigate treatment. The various other measurements of haemoglobin level, such as mean corpuscular haemoglobin (MCV) and mean cell haemoglobin (MCH), help to identify a possible cause for the anaemia

- Low haemoglobin levels in young women are most often due to heavy periods. Low haemoglobin can also be due to the inherited condition thalassaemia

- High haemoglobin can be caused by smoking or a medical condition that increases the amount of red cells produced, called polycythaemia rubra vera

Haemoglobin		
	Normal	Significantly low
Males	> 13.2 g/dl	< 12 g/dl
Females	11.5 g/dl	< 11 g/dl

Platelets

- Platelets are required for blood clotting; too low levels can lead to excessive bleeding, whereas too high levels can lead to blood clotting

Platelet count
Normal range: 150–400

White cell count

- The white cell count is very similar in men and women, and remains fairly constant throughout life

Total white cell count
Normal range: 4–11 $\times$ 10^9/l

- *High white cell counts* > 11.0 can be caused by smoking, infection, pregnancy, gout, haematological cancers (e.g. leukaemia) and by taking some prescribed medications such as prednisolone, digoxin and lithium

- *Low white cell counts* < 4.0 can be caused by infections, particularly viral and other infections such as tuberculosis, as well as some drugs, especially disease-modifying drugs used in rheumatology, such as sulphasalazine, methotrexate and leflunamide

BOX 29.3   Biochemical tests

Liver function tests

- Raised levels of bilirubin occur in jaundice. Urine testing may be helpful (see Figure 29.1). Liver function blood tests and an abdominal ultrasound examination will determine the likely cause of the jaundice

Bilirubin
Normal range: < 36 mmol/l

Liver enzymes

- Raised liver enzyme measurements suggest liver disease and vary according to the cause, which may be gallbladder disease, hepatitis or cancer

Alkaline phosphatase
Normal range: 90–300 IU/l

Aspartate transaminase (ALT)
Normal range: < 50 IU/l

Alanine aminotransferase (AST)
Normal range: < 45 IU/l

Gamma-glutamyl transferase (GGT)		
	Males	Females
Normal range	> 70 IU/l	> 40 IU/l

Uric acid

- Uric acid levels are raised in gout

Uric acid		
	Males	Females
Normal range	< 420 mmol/l	< 360 mmol/l

Urea and electrolytes

- Abnormalities of renal function occur in renal disease

Sodium
Normal range: 135–145 mmol/l

Potassium
Normal range: 3.5–5.3 mmol/l

Creatinine
Normal range: 60–120 mmol/l

Urea
Normal range: < 8.5 mmol/l

Blood sugar

- A fasting level of 6-7 mmol/l indicates impaired glucose metabolism and a further test is necessary
- A fasting blood sugar level of > 7 mmol/l suggests diabetes, and a further test or oral glucose tolerance test may be required

Blood sugar
Normal range, fasting: 3.5–5.5 mmol/l

Chapter 30

Venepuncture

Sharon Harris and Steven Walker

Venepuncture is an essential skill for practice nurses. For many, taking blood is a routine and enjoyable part of their job. For the novice, however, it can seem very daunting. Do not panic – we all felt this way once. Like all skills, it requires training, preparation and practice, and it becomes steadily easier with experience.[1] Usually, venepuncture is straightforward, but it can be difficult, and on occasions even the most experienced practitioner is defeated and has to seek help.

INDICATIONS

Venepuncture simply means inserting a needle into a vein. Indications are listed in Box 30.1. As a practice nurse, your role will be confined to taking blood for subsequent laboratory analysis. Usually, the request will have originated from one of the doctors in the surgery. Alternatively, the patient may be undergoing routine screening or regular monitoring, as with measuring the international normalized ratio (INR) in patients receiving warfarin therapy.

CONTRAINDICATIONS

Venepuncture is generally a safe procedure with few complications. It is not contraindicated in patients with infections, even human immuno-

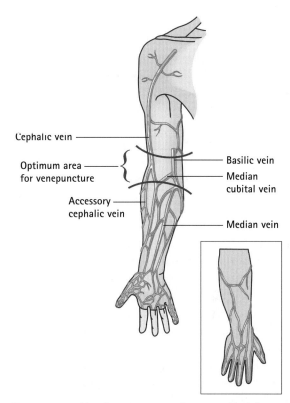

Figure 30.1   Venous anatomy at the antecubital fossa.

deficiency virus (HIV) or hepatitis B, or in those with clotting defects such as haemophilia or those receiving warfarin treatment. The universal precautions and care taken when carrying out venepuncture in any patient will be sufficient to protect against cross-infection and other complications such as haematoma and bruising. Routine blood testing in anaemic subjects will not appreciably affect their condition.

CHOOSING A SUITABLE VEIN

In adults, the best veins to use are the cephalic or basilic veins in the front of the arm, over the elbow crease (antecubital fossa). Here, the veins usually have an H-shaped arrangement (Figure 30.1) and are relatively large. Once a tourniquet is applied, they can usually be both seen and felt. Where possible, use the non-dominant arm – if the patient is right-handed, take blood from the left arm. This is not a hard and fast rule; go for whichever side is the best, especially when learning. Try to succeed first time. Avoid puncturing fibrosed, inflamed or fragile veins. It is also preferable to avoid an injured arm and the side affected by a stroke or surgery/radiotherapy, as may be found after mastectomy.

An alternative is to select a vein on the back of the hand (see Figure 30.1) or the cephalic vein on the thumb side of the wrist. Possible disadvantages are that the vessels at these sites are more mobile and tend to collapse. A useful tip is to insert a smaller 'butterfly' needle; this can still be attached to a vacuum system.

EQUIPMENT

Make sure you have everything to hand before you start (Box 30.2). Rummaging around for a swab half way through looks unprofessional, and if you move you may damage the vein.

Wearing protection will not prevent a needlestick injury, but can reduce the risk of coming into contact with potentially infected blood and helps to prevent cross-infection. Any nurse who is required to carry out venepuncture as part of his or her role should be aware of local policies and procedures regarding needlestick injuries. Patients may feel that use of such protection is insulting and intimidating, but a

> **BOX 30.2   Equipment for venepuncture**
>
> - Disposable gloves and apron (plus protective eyewear when dealing with HIV and hepatitis subjects)
> - Tourniquet
> - Alcohol swabs
> - Vacutainer and Vacutainer needle
> - Sharps box
> - Gauze and sticking plaster
> - The correct request forms

simple factual explanation usually helps. Unfortunately, wearing gloves makes feeling for the vein more difficult.

The best type of tourniquet is broad with a quick-release mechanism. The old-fashioned rubber tube tourniquets are more likely to pinch the skin and cause local trauma, including nerve damage. Infection at the puncture site is very rare. Prevention by rubbing the skin with alcohol wipes is of no proven benefit, but has become part of tradition. The experienced patient may question your ability if you do not use one.

Anaesthetic

Some subjects may ask for local anaesthetic. Explain that an injectable agent such as 1% lignocaine will obscure the vein and cause further discomfort. Also, the patient will have to suffer two puncture wounds, not one. Topical anaesthetic creams such as Emla applied 30 minutes before taking blood are effective and may be useful, especially in children or the squeamish.

PREPARATION

The secret is in the preparation. Make sure the patient is sitting or lying comfortably. A couch is safer for those at risk of fainting. Talk to the patient and put him or her at ease. This may provide the opportunity to give advice and further help. You can be preparing your equipment in a business-like way at the same time, and this will inspire confidence. Ask the patient to roll up their sleeve as high as possible. Support the arm on a couch or work surface. You may find performing venepuncture easier if you are sitting down. Make sure the area is well illuminated.

Apply the tourniquet above the elbow and ask the patient to open and close his or her fist vigorously. After about 30–60 seconds, the main veins should be sufficiently engorged to see and feel. Where the veins are poor, examine the opposite side and backs of the hands.

Attach the needle to a vacuum system blood bottle if you are using one. It twists in like fitting a light bulb.

PROCEDURE

- Fix the vein by pulling down on the skin just below the venepuncture site, or, with a vein on the back of the hand, by bending the wrist (Figure 30.2).
- Insert the needle (bevel uppermost) confidently at 30–45° to the skin and into the vein in one smooth movement.
- You may feel the vein wall 'give'.
- Once in the vein, advance the tip a short distance. If you are using a syringe, steady the

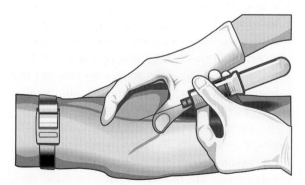

Figure 30.2   Venepuncture being performed.

needle and pull back on the plunger until you have sufficient blood. Otherwise, unscrew the vacuum bottle while stabilizing the needle and attach the next one within 1 minute if you need to.

- Release and remove the tourniquet – you would be surprised how often this gets forgotten.
- Place a cotton wool ball over the venepuncture site (an alcohol swab stings) and only then remove the needle.
- Ask the patient to press firmly on the site for at least 1 minute, and usually longer in anti-coagulated subjects or those with clotting abnormalities.
- Apply a sticking plaster.
- Dispose of the needle in a sharps box.
- Occasionally, you may have difficulties. Box 30.3 gives you advice on when to call for help.

COMPLICATIONS

Pain and bruising

Pain and bruising are the most common problems and are minimized by a practised and confident technique (Box 30.4). Continuous direct pressure

---

over the venepuncture site, after the needle has been withdrawn, helps reduce bruising.

Missing the vein

When trying to puncture a mobile vein, especially in elderly subjects, the needle sometimes passes along the outside of the vessel and fails to enter the lumen. Try pulling firmly downwards on the skin to straighten and stabilize the vein. Another trick is to aim for the junction where two veins meet, or use a 'butterfly' needle. Some more tips are provided in Box 30.5.

Piercing the back wall of the vein

This is common when starting out. Apart from causing a bruise, coming through the other side of the vein is not serious. The trick is, once you get

---

> **BOX 30.3   When to call for help**
>
> - Small children have small veins. Also, they tend to wriggle about a lot and scream. Unless you are experienced, leave them to someone else[3]
> - If you cannot see or feel any veins anywhere, despite all the tricks, get someone else and stay around to watch how they deal with the situation
> - If you have unsuccessfully tried two or three times, call for assistance – it is unlikely you are going to succeed on this occasion
> - Avoid carrying out any procedures on your family and friends

---

> **BOX 30.4   Keeping out of trouble**
>
> - Always explain to the patient what you are about to do and why. Ask them if they understand and are happy for you to continue (verbal consent). You do not at present require a signed consent form for routine phlebotomy
> - Make absolutely sure that if the patient has hearing difficulties or speaks little English, they are really the patient referred to on the form
> - In dialysis patients, avoid the arteriovenous fistula arm and never use the fistula. Liase with the dialysis unit, who will usually take the blood for you if a form is provided
> - Until you are more experienced, avoid phlebotomy in children and those with poor veins. If you cannot see or feel any suitable veins, you are likely to miss. Take your time. Poking around with a needle is not good practice. With experience, you will find that palpation will often reveal large deep veins that you may not be able to see

blood in your syringe, immediately change the angle of advance so your needle is directed along the lumen of the vessel. Occasionally, it is possible to retrieve the situation by gently pulling back, but often you have to start again.

Trauma and infection

Causing a clot in the vein (thrombosis), inflammation/infection (phlebitis) or both (thrombophlebitis) are uncommon after routine phlebotomy and are rarely serious. You are very unlikely to advance the needle so far as to damage muscle, arteries, nerves or bone. You should, however, be familiar with the anatomy of the region, so that you can be sure to avoid these related structures.

Blood bottles and request forms

Common tests are checking the patient's full blood count (FBC), urea and electrolytes (U&Es), liver function tests (LFTs), fasting blood sugar (BS),

---

BOX 30.5   Venepuncture tips

1. Politely request any friends/relatives/small children to take a seat outside or behind the curtain
2. Tricks to fill the veins include hanging the hand as low as possible, a brief period of exercise, or putting the arm in a basin of warm water
3. One of the authors (who does not enjoy being the subject of this procedure) finds it helpful to squeeze his upper arm during phlebotomy to mask the pain from the needle site
4. Leaving the tourniquet on beyond a couple of minutes causes pain and dusky discoloration, which makes visualizing the veins increasingly difficult
5. If there is swelling and pain, remove the needle quickly and apply pressure to the area to minimize trauma

---

cholesterol and clotting. Each requires a different, colour-coded blood bottle.

The bottles require a gentle shake after filling to ensure that any anticoagulant or preservative is properly mixed with the blood.

In most clinical areas, there will be a chart to help you choose the correct tubes. Label the blood bottles either before you take the sample or immediately afterwards and keep them together with the forms, equipment and any patient records. Using a tray aids safety.

Do not deal with more than one patient at a time. Store the samples and send to the laboratory as soon as possible, because delays may affect the results.

VENEPUNCTURE AND PROFESSIONAL PRACTICE

Many practice nurses have performed venepuncture during their training or hospital career. If you are a little rusty or are completely new to this, get some training.

There may be local courses. These generally involve lectures on safe practice and practical sessions using an orange, rubber model arm complete with artificial blood or taking blood from each other. In your practice, ask a more experienced colleague to be your mentor. He or she can guide you during your early procedures.

Venepuncture will be a routine part of your job, but is still an extended role, so it is up to you to ensure that you are adequately trained and experienced to carry out the procedure safely.[2]

SUMMARY

Venepuncture is a routine part of the activities of a practice nurse. You will be required to take blood for a variety of diagnostic, monitoring and screening purposes. This chapter stresses safe practice, good communication and prior preparation. It is essential that you have received adequate training, that your practice has been supervised and assessed and that you maintain your proficiency.

ESSENTIAL SKILLS

- Put the patient at ease
- Be well organized to give an air of confidence and professionalism
- Do not take on venepuncture in more difficult cases until you have experience of easier ones

REFERENCES

1. Black F, Hughes J. Venepuncture. Nursing Standard 1997; 11(41): 49–55.
2. Nursing and Midwifery Council. Code of Professional Conduct. London: Nursing and Midwifery Council, 2002.
3. Willock J, Richardson J, Brazier A, Powell C, Mitchell E. Peripheral venepuncture in infants and children. Nursing Standard 2004; 18(27): 43–50, 52, 55.

Section 4

Management and professional issues

Obtaining a valid consent

Bridgit Dimond

Before carrying out any procedure or treatment on a patient, the practice nurse must first obtain a valid consent. Never assume that consent has already been given, even if the patient has discussed the treatment with the GP. This chapter examines the legal issues that apply to consent in adults; the position for children is discussed in Chapter 1.

TRESPASS TO THE PERSON

Consent is required from a mentally competent adult in order to prevent any interference with his or her person. To be valid it must be given voluntarily, without fraud or coercion. The absence of consent, when the patient has the necessary competence to give it, could lead to an action for trespass to the person (also called battery). In such an action, the claimant must show that a procedure was carried out for which he or she did not give consent. It is not necessary to show that any harm occurred, as even if the patient benefited, the unauthorized treatment constitutes trespass.

In the highly publicized case of Miss B, who asked the court for her ventilator to be switched off, the only issue before the court was whether she had the necessary mental competence to give valid consent.[1] When this was established by medical evidence, the judge had no option in law other than to hold that the switching off of the ventilator would be lawful and that a trespass to her person had been committed when she was placed on the ventilator against her will.

THE DUTY OF CARE TO INFORM

An action for breach of the duty of care to inform relies upon the claimant being able to show that the health professional failed to inform him or her of information that related to a significant risk of substantial harm. A patient who suffers significant side-effects from a treatment and had not been told about the possibility of that harm can argue that there was a breach of the duty of care to inform.

In 2004 the House of Lords heard a case that determined that the claimant is required to prove that they would not have agreed to treatment had they known of those side-effects.[2]

APPLICATION OF THE LAW

Trespass to the person

With regard to the situation laid out in Box 31.1 it would appear that Mary is mentally competent. It will be a question of evidence as to what exactly was said between them before the ear syringing was done. If Yvonne can show that Mary agreed to the ear syringing and that she did not hold herself out as being a doctor, then it could be argued that Mary gave a valid consent to the treatment. In any court case Mary would have the burden of proving on a balance of probabilities that she believed Yvonne to be a doctor and therefore she did not give a valid consent.

Duty of care to inform

Even if Mary did give consent and therefore could not succeed in a trespass to the person action, she

---

BOX 31.1   Situation 1

Consent for ear syringing
Yvonne Davis, a practice nurse who is qualified to undertake ear syringing, is asked by the GP to syringe the ears of Mary Brown who is 47 years old. The client consents to the procedure and Yvonne carries it out, but unfortunately Mary subsequently complains that she is deaf and claims that this is the result of the ear syringing. She also says that she would not have agreed to her ears being syringed if she had known that a nurse would be carrying out the procedure, and therefore she did not give consent. What is the law?

The situation gives rise to several different legal issues:
- Did Mary give a valid consent?
- If so, how (if at all) should the consent have been evidenced?
- Is the deafness a risk of ear syringing?
- What should the practice nurse have told Mary?
- Did the practice nurse follow the correct procedure in carrying out the treatment?

---

may argue that Yvonne failed to provide her with essential information about the treatment. She would have to prove that any reasonable practitioner would have informed her of the risk of deafness, that the deafness was caused by the ear syringing, and that Yvonne's failure to inform her was therefore a breach of her duty of care. The House of Lords in the Sidaway case held that deciding what information should be conveyed to the patient prior to treatment depended on the reasonable standard of profes-sional practice at that time.[3] This is grounded in the Bolam test that implies that practitioners be judged against a backcloth of their peers.[4]

Evidence of the consent

In law the essential fact is that the patient understands in general terms what is to be done and gives a valid consent to that procedure. Consent could be given by word of mouth, in writing or even by non-verbal behaviour, for example rolling up a sleeve, opening one's mouth for the temperature to be taken. All of these are valid in law, but it is clear that their value as evidence varies considerably. As Situation 1 illustrates, there is considerable advantage in obtaining evidence of consent in writing.

The Department of Health (DoH) has provided guidance on the law relating to consent and its implementation and provides forms.[5, 6] Had Yvonne made use of these forms as evidence that Mary agreed to the ear syringing and that she was notified of risks, the dispute may not have arisen. The forms can be used by any health professional, including practice nurses. Form 1 is for procedures to be carried out on an adult patient. Form 3 is for procedures to be carried out where the patient does not lose consciousness. The forms enable the health professional to identify the treatment that is to be given and outline the benefits and risks that have been explained to the patient. The patient then signs that they understand the benefits and risks, are aware of who may carry out the treatment, and that they wish to proceed. This would have prevented any misunderstanding over whether Mary wanted the procedure to be carried out specifically by a doctor.

A MENTALLY INCAPACITATED ADULT

Where an adult is incapable of giving consent then action can be carried out of necessity, without consent, in the best interests of that person. The legal basis for this (in England, Wales and Northern Ireland) is a decision of the House of Lords (i.e. the common law or judge-made law as opposed to a statute). In Scotland the Adult with Incapacity (Scotland) Act 2000 came into force on 2 April 2002.

In the case of Re F, the House of Lords heard an application for the sterilization of a woman with severe mental disabilities who was incapable of

giving consent, and declared that an operation could be performed in her best interests.[7] Applying this to Situation 2 (Box 31.2), where Yvonne was caring for Mary's mother who lacked the mental competence to make decisions, Yvonne would obviously discuss the proposed treatment with Mary, but Mary does not have the right in law to consent to or refuse treatment on her mother's behalf. If Yvonne considers that the treatment is in Mary's mother's best interests, then she can give it.

However, the Court of Appeal overturned a decision permitting the sterilization of another adult patient S, who was incapable of giving consent.[8]

If Yvonne uses Form 4 in the DoH's guidance she would be required to identify the reason for the patient's mental incapacity, and state the proposed treatment and the risks and benefits associated with it. Mary as a relative could sign that she understands that her mother is mentally incapacitated and that the proposed treatment is in her best interests. In determining what

---

Box 31.2   Situation 2

A mentally incapacitated adult: ear syringing
Yvonne Davis, a practice nurse who is qualified to undertake ear syringing, is asked by the GP to syringe the ears of Mary Brown's mother who is 85 years old. Yvonne carries out the procedure, but unfortunately Mary subsequently complains that her mother has become deaf and claims that this is the result of the ear syringing. She also says that her mother did not give consent to the ears being syringed. What is the law?

What would be the law if the above situation arose: i.e. if, instead of Mary receiving the ear syringing, she had brought to the surgery her elderly mother of 85 who suffered from Alzheimer's and was incapable of giving consent, but who had been seen by a GP who recommended ear syringing as being in her best interests?

treatment is in the patient's best interests the health professional would have to take into account significant risks of substantial harm associated with that treatment.

CONCLUSION

The two scenarios discussed here assume that Yvonne acted within her professional competence and carried out the procedures according to the reasonable standard of professional practice. If this were not so, then other legal issues would arise. This chapter has dealt with only a small part

of the law on consent, and practitioners who are interested in following up this topic might find *The Legal Aspects of Consent*[9] of assistance.

ESSENTIAL SKILLS

- Understand what constitutes a valid consent
- Obtain consent for all procedures/treatments, or act in the best interests of a mentally incapacitated adult who is unable to give consent
- Recognize when consent has been given
- Give patients all the information they need in order to give a valid consent

REFERENCES

1. B (consent to treatment capacity) Re v An NHS Hospital Trust. 26 March 2002; [2002] 2 ALL ER 449.
2. Chester v Afshar. Times Law Report 13 June 2002. [2002] 3 ALL ER 552 CA.
3. Sidaway v Bethlem Royal Hospital Governors and Others. [1985] 1 ALL ER 643; [1985] AC 871.
4. Bolam v Friern Hospital Management Committee; [1957] 2 ALL ER.
5. Department of Health. Reference Guide to Consent for Examination or Treatment. London: DoH, 2001. Available at: http://www.dh.gov.uk
6. Department of Health. Good Practice in Consent Implementation Guide. London: DoH; 2001.
7. F v West Berkshire HA & Another. [1989] 2 ALL ER 545; [1990] 2 AC 1.
8. Re S (Adult Patient: Sterilisation: Patient's Best Interests). Also known as: Re SL (Adult Patient) (Medical Treatment) and as Re SL v SL. [2001] Fam 15; [2000] 3 WLR 1288; [2000] 2 FLR 389; (2000) 55 BMLR 105 (CA).
9. Dimond, B. The Legal Aspects of Consent Dinton: Quay Books, 2003.

Chapter 32

Infection control

Keith Hampton

Standard precautions of infection control are wide-ranging principles that aim to reduce the risk of disease transmission in healthcare settings, even when the source of infection is not known or obvious. It is essential for anyone new to practice nursing to review the standard precautions in use in the primary care setting as outlined in this chapter.

HAND HYGIENE

To maximize hand-washing compliance correct facilities should be available for practice staff and patients to decontaminate their hands. Sinks for hand washing should be reserved for this purpose and not shared with other activities such as washing instruments. They should be equipped with lever-operated mixer taps to ensure that water is at a comfortable temperature. A good liquid soap should be available, preferably in a wall-mounted dispenser.

Washing hands well at the right time is more important than the agent used or the length of time taken.[1] The ideal technique should be quick, cover all surfaces of the hands, reduce hand contamination to the lowest possible level and be free from noticeable side-effects.[2] Quality products and a good technique will help to maintain skin condition, but these can be supplemented by the use of emollients in a wall-mounted or free-standing dispenser. Communal tubs are easily contaminated and should be avoided.

Good quality, paper hand towels in a wall-mounted dispenser should be available for drying hands. Cloth and terry towels are not suitable for the surgery as they are quickly contaminated and can act as a reservoir.[3, 4] A foot-operated waste bin will ensure that hand towels can be disposed of without recontaminating the hands. Hand rubs and gels with alcohol are a convenient means of decontaminating the hands when not visibly soiled and should be available in all clinical areas.

PERSONAL PROTECTIVE EQUIPMENT

An employer has a duty to ensure that personal protective equipment is always readily available, free of charge, where risk cannot be controlled by other means.[5] Before undertaking any task an assessment should be made of the likelihood of the healthcare worker's clothing, skin, conjunctivae or mucous membranes becoming contaminated with blood, body fluids, secretions and excretions (Figure 32.1).

Gloves

Hands have a key role in the transmission of infection and gloves can reduce the number of micro-organisms acquired. However, hands should still be washed when gloves are removed. Gloves must always be changed between caring for different patients, or between different activities for the same patient.[6] They should be discarded after use, as clinical waste, and never be washed or re-used. Gloves should bear the CE mark indicating that the product complies with European directives on safety and performance.

The examination glove is the type needed most often in surgery. Powder-free latex remains the material of choice, as it affords the best protection against blood, body fluids and blood-borne viruses. Examination gloves may be sterile, for performing aseptic procedures, or non-sterile for other procedures involving blood or body fluids.

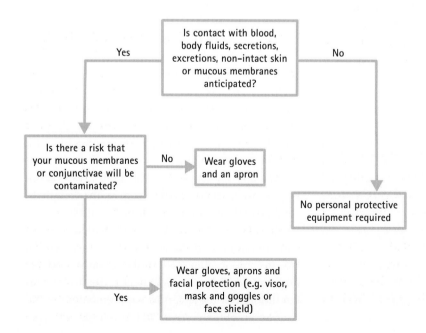

Figure 32.1 Personal protective equipment risk assessment.

Sterile surgical gloves should be available if surgical procedures are undertaken in the practice. Alternatives to latex, such as nitrile and neoprene, can be used if staff or patients are sensitive to latex. If you have a reaction to any latex product you should seek the advice of an occupational health department or your GP.

Aprons

A plastic apron should be worn when exposure to blood or body fluids is anticipated, when clothing may become wet or when there is direct contact with a known infectious patient.

Plastic aprons are single-use items and should be discarded, as clinical waste, on completion of a task.

Masks, eye protection and face shields

Masks protect both patients and staff from micro-organisms. They should be worn when blood, or any other body fluid, may contaminate the mucous membranes of the mouth. Eye protection can be goggles (worn in combination with a mask), a face shield (a single-use mask with built-in plastic eye shield) or a full-face plastic visor. One of these options should be worn if there is a risk of eyes being contaminated with blood, other body fluids or chemicals.

WASTE DISPOSAL

A practice has a 'cradle to grave' responsibility for the waste it produces. The practice should ensure that only licensed contractors are engaged to remove waste from the premises for disposal, and also that clinical waste is transported in suitable, approved, rigid packaging.[7] All waste bags and sharps boxes should be labelled with the practice details so that any waste can be traced back to source if necessary.

Waste bags should comply with the national colour-coding system of yellow bags for clinical waste and black bags for household-type waste. Nothing sharp, or potentially sharp, such as glass, should ever be placed in a waste bag. These items should be placed in cardboard collection boxes, as should aerosols, which can explode if incinerated.

SHARPS SAFETY

Injuries resulting from sharps contaminated with blood or other high-risk body fluids can have serious or even fatal consequences for healthcare workers. All sharps, but particularly used ones, should be handled as little as possible and never passed from hand to hand. Needles should never be resheathed or disconnected from syringes, but discarded together as one unit. Dispose of sharps in an approved, correctly assembled, sharps container at the point of use. The container should be sited below eye level, but not on the floor or in other locations where children may have access. Sharps containers should never be overfilled, but locked prior to final disposal when two-thirds full.

EXPOSURE TO BLOOD AND BODY FLUIDS

Healthcare employers, including GPs, must ensure that arrangements are in place for the management of exposure to blood-borne viruses and other micro-organisms. This can occur percutaneously (e.g. sharp instruments or bites that break the skin), by contamination of non-intact skin (cuts, abrasions or eczematous skin), or by contamination of the conjunctivae or the mucous membranes of the mouth.

First aid for a percutaneous injury consists of encouraging the wound to bleed (do not suck the wound), washing under running water and the application of a waterproof dressing. Rinse or irrigate with plenty of cold water in cases of contamination of non-intact skin, mucous membranes or conjunctivae. Incident forms should be completed in accordance with local policy and expert help sought – from the occupational health department, consultant microbiologist, infection-control doctor or consultant in communicable disease control – so that an urgent risk assessment can be undertaken. Make a point of finding out the name and contact details of the relevant person in your area as soon as possible.

Spillages of blood and other body fluids can be conveniently dealt with by using a proprietary spill kit. These contain everything necessary to deal with a spill, but they usually contain chlorine-releasing products, making them unsuitable for use on carpets and on urine spills.

SPECIMEN COLLECTION

Specimens should be collected into an appropriate leak-proof container – usually supplied by the laboratory processing the specimen. Remove any contamination from the outside of the container, then put it in a double-sleeved, plastic specimen bag. Put the completed request form in the other pocket of the bag. This ensures that even if the specimen leaks it should be contained within the bag and the form is protected. Check that whoever collects specimens from the practice transports them in a strong, leak-proof box. This should be made of an impervious, easily cleaned material and labelled to indicate the biohazard inside.

DECONTAMINATION

Decontamination is no less important in general practice than elsewhere, particularly with more minor surgery being carried out in primary care. The risk category of each item must be assessed to determine the appropriate decontamination method (i.e. cleaning, disinfection or sterilization).

Low-risk items, such as stethoscopes, do not come into contact with patients or only touch their intact skin. This type of equipment must be cleaned or disinfected after use. Intermediate risk items, such as vaginal examination specula, come into contact with intact skin or mucous membranes. These items do not need to be sterile at the point of use but they must have been cleaned and sterilized between uses and stored in clean conditions.[8]

High-risk items – such as surgical instruments and specula used for intrauterine procedures – penetrate the skin, come into contact with non-intact skin or mucous membranes or enter a normally sterile area of the body. These instruments must be sterile at the point of use.

Equipment

Mechanical cleaning equipment, such as washer-disinfectors or ultrasonic baths, are preferable to manual cleaning. They are efficient, and results are reproducible and can be validated.[9] This equipment should be operated in accordance with the NHS Health Technical Memorandum (HTM) 2030.[10]

If cleaning instruments manually, personal protective equipment should be worn and a designated area available. This should contain a sink that is not used for washing hands and that allows submersion of instruments. High standards of cleaning are an essential prerequisite to disinfection and sterilization.

A benchtop steam sterilizer (BSS) is frequently used for sterilizing instruments. The most common type is the gravity displacement BSS, but these models are not suitable for hollow devices, those with lumens or for any wrapped loads (i.e. in pouches). They should be operated in accordance with the Medical Devices Agency Bulletin 2002 (06) and HTM 2031.[11, 12] The former document requires daily, weekly, quarterly and annual tests to be completed and recorded in a log book. The HTM 2031 document covers the provision of steam that is free from impurities and details how the water reservoir should be maintained.

The practice should consider alternative decontamination options such as presterilized, single-use items, which should never be re-used, or the use of a local sterile services department (SSD) if available. The cost per instrument is generally cheaper than reprocessing on practice premises and all legal responsibility remains with the SSD.[8]

CONCLUSION

Practice nurses have skills learned in different healthcare settings. The need for good hand hygiene, correct use of personal protective equipment, sharps safety and specimen collection are common to all areas of practice. However instrument decontamination, disposal of the practice's waste and sources of help following exposure to blood and body fluids may be new considerations.

ESSENTIAL SKILLS

- Effective hand hygiene procedures
- Knowledge of full range of personal protective equipment available and when to use it
- Ability to ensure appropriate waste disposal
- Effective sharps safety procedures to prevent needlestick injury
- Ability to manage exposure to blood and body fluids according to local policy and knowledge of whom to report incidents to
- Ability to ensure safe and secure collection and transport of specimens
- Knowledge of equipment decontamination procedures and their use according to appropriate risk levels

---

REFERENCES

1. Ayliffe GAJ, Fraise AP, Geddes AM, Mitchell K. Control of Hospital Infection. A Practical Handbook, 4th edn. London: Arnold, 2000.
2. Pittet D, Boyce JM. Hand hygiene and patient care: pursuing the Semmelweis legacy. Lancet Infectious Diseases 2001; 1: 9–20.
3. Infection Control Nurses Association. Hand Decontamination Guidelines. London: ICNA/Regent, 2002.
4. McCulloch J, Finn L, Bowell B. Management of known infections. In: McCulloch J (ed.). Infection Control: Science Management and Practice. London: Whurr, 2000.
5. The Personal Protective Equipment at Work Regulations, 1992. Statutory Instrument 1992 No. 2966. London: HMSO, 1992.
6. Department of Health. The epic project: developing national evidence-based guidelines for preventing healthcare associated infections. J Hosp Infect 2001; 47: S1–S82.
7. Health & Safety Commission, Health Services Advisory Committee. Safe Disposal of Clinical Waste. London: HSE Books, 1999.
8. Community Infection Control Nurses Network, Royal College of General Practitioners. Infection Control Guidance for General Practice. Bathgate: Infection Control Nurses Association, 2003.
9. NHS Estates. A Protocol for the Local Decontamination of Surgical Instruments. London: NHS Estates, 2001
10. NHS Estates. Washer-disinfectors. Management Policy, Health Technical Memorandum 2030. London: HMSO, 1995
11. Medical Devices Agency. Benchtop steam sterilizers – guidance on purchase, operation and maintenance. MDA DB2002(06). London: Medical Devices Agency, 2002.
12. NHS Estates. Clean Steam for Sterilization. Health Technical Memorandum 2031. London: HMSO, 1997.

Chapter 33

Child protection

Briony Ladbury

CHAPTER CONTENTS

The report (2003) into the truly dreadful death of 8-year-old Victoria Climbié is finally beginning to have an impact. The conclusions reached in the Laming Report that the child-protection systems failed her spectacularly have been widely accepted.[1] In the report Lord Laming expresses dismay about the low priority that child protection assumed and amazement that, without exception, none of the professionals in any of the agencies involved had the 'presence of mind' to follow what he described as 'relatively straightforward procedures'.

The message running through the report is that the systems to protect children developed over the last decade are basically sound, but the actual practice by those directly delivering services leaves a lot to be desired. Accountability and communication were also judged to be flawed. Lord Laming speaks of an 'organizational malaise' with regard to protecting children that is so widespread that the responsibility for the death of Victoria needs to be shared evenly between senior managers, service managers and practitioners at field level.

THE IMPACT OF THE LAMING INQUIRY

The Laming Report has made an impact on the way we practise. It was an important influence on the Government's green paper *Every Child Matters*, which was published in September 2003.[2]

Health practitioners, largely those working in the acute hospital setting, were heavily criticized in the Victoria Climbié Inquiry, but it is also fair to say that the primary healthcare teams involved invited some criticism too, pinpointing an apparent lack of child-centred practice. Victoria's new-patient assessment on initial registration with a GP surgery showed little evidence of the practice nurse engaging with Victoria, and this invisibility was mirrored when the family changed their doctor. Unfortunately, the new practice registered Victoria without seeing her at all.

Many of the longer term health recommendations in the Laming Report were implemented in January 2005, and allude to the development of child protection practice within the primary healthcare team. In short, practitioners working in primary healthcare teams will need to be pro-active in exercising their child-protection responsibilities, and performance monitoring of child-protection practice will be undertaken more rigorously in the future.

CHANGING CULTURES AND REALITIES

The pace of change in primary care has been unrelenting. A highly skilled workforce is needed to meet the increasing demands from the public and politicians. Primary care workers must feel that they are being asked to be masters of everything.

Child protection is an area of work that is hard to contemplate. It is highly complex and can have serious consequences for children, families, communities and professionals alike. It is not unusual for some practitioners to feel out of their depth and anxious when a child presents with child-protection issues. Nevertheless, practice nurses will inevitably be faced at some time with a case that raises child-protection concerns.

All too often there are accounts of concerns being identified but ignored, or identified but not recorded, or recorded in a way that minimizes the level of risk observed. Situations that seriously impact on children are therefore not coming to the attention of the authorities at a stage where intervention could have prevented a child from suffering significant harm.

In my experience, this poor practice is not so much about practitioners wanting to sweep difficult issues under the carpet, but more about the need for training and support in order that staff can achieve a competency level whereby they can trust their intuition, analyse their observations and be confident about when to seek advice about triggering action.

Practice nurses must be skilled in engaging with and responding to children in need of support or protection. This can only be brought about by appropriate training, supervision, professional support and protocols that can provide a feeling of safety in an area of work that cuts deeply into the values and subconscious processes of the practitioner, and that will by its very nature trigger an interference in what is, after all, somebody else's private family life.

Not so long ago the health visitor was considered a central and expert figure for child-protection practice, to the extent that health visitors may have been prepared to make third-party referrals on behalf of other members of the primary healthcare team. This is no longer seen as good practice, particularly since the model of health visiting in many places has changed from a service that afforded routine visiting to all children under 5 years old, to one of a targeted service. *Every Child Matters* recommends a return to universal services and a focus on prevention, but this is likely to take some time to establish and robust services need to be in place during any period of reorganization.[2]

The frequent universal monitoring of all children coupled with the broad knowledge of individual family dynamics and circumstances has not been the working norm for many modern health visitors. Over-reliance on the health visitor is therefore often not in a child's best interests. It is now very likely that the practice nurse will be the first to engage with a family and that the GP practice will be the starting point for following through child protection concerns. It is, however, essential and still good practice to share information with colleagues, and much can be gleaned from a discussion with others who may be actively working with the family in another capacity.

However, practice nurses must act within their own accountability framework and take full responsibility for identifying and referring children who are in need or at risk. This level of involvement requires a professional confidence that enables a practitioner to make decisions, challenge the opinions of colleagues and seek expert advice where there is uncertainty.

The most recent edition of a multi-agency practice document *Working Together to Safeguard Children* issued in 1999 is the main practice document to which all professional guidelines adhere.[3] Within its pages, a paragraph alluding to primary healthcare teams states that they 'are well placed to recognize when a child is potentially in need of extra help or services to promote health and development, or is at risk of harm'.

Chapter 5 of this same guidance entitled *Handling Individual Cases* was considered post-Laming to be falling short of achieving its aim in practice, and a new document called *What To Do if You're Worried a Child is Being Abused* was hurried into print.[4] In June 2003, a summary, in the form of a booklet, was posted to every registered nurse in England and Wales. The booklet contains useful practical advice and outlines child-protection practice in a series of easy to follow flow charts. If you do not have a copy, you can get one free from the Department of Health (DoH) publications office.

At about the same time the new Royal College of Nursing guidelines were issued. The launch in June 2002 of *Child Protection: Every Nurse's Responsibility* promoted the message that all nurses have a professional and personal responsibility to be able to spot the signs of child abuse and know how to take action.[5] The guidance, however, also outlines the responsibilities of primary care trusts (PCTs) and other employers to enable nurses to practise safely.

CHILD PROTECTION IN PRACTICE

Practice nurses are not child-protection specialists and it is essential that they are supported in their child-protection practice and are able to call on an expert to assist them with any aspect of child-protection work. There are, however, some practical skills that are fundamental to child protection.

The Framework for the Assessment of Children in Need and their Families was published in 2000.[6] The conceptual framework outlines how anyone, including health professionals, working with children should undertake an assessment of a child. The framework consists of a triangular structure, the sides of which represent the three mainstays in terms of child development (Figure 33.1). Within the triangle is a circle symbolizing child-centred practice. The three 'domains' – child development, family and environmental factors, and parenting capacity – are considered essential components for the growth and welfare of children.

The domains are then subdivided into 'dimensions' to help practitioners view the child in an ecological and holistic context. To summarize,

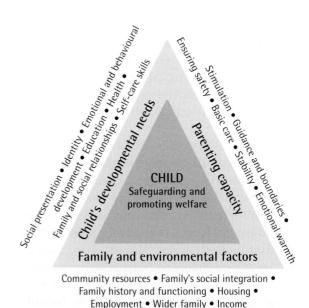

Figure 33.1 The framework for the assessment of children in need and their families (2000). Reproduced with permission of the Department of Health.

practitioners are urged to view a child in terms of these three important areas of his or her life. This simple but effective assessment tool brings into focus the factors that can impact adversely on the welfare of a child. Parenting capacity is in itself an area which may be all too evident in the GP surgery. Children can suffer greatly in families where there is drug or alcohol abuse, unstable mental illness or domestic violence.

Vulnerable adults falling into these categories are highly likely to use primary healthcare services, and many will care for children. Practice nurses who suspect emotional abuse or neglect of children caused by poor parenting have a duty to act in the child's best interest and with the same conviction as when a child presents with an obvious inflicted physical injury.

GETTING THE HISTORY RIGHT

History taking is the single most important part of sound child-protection practice. Basic patient details are extremely important and should be recorded in full at the earliest possible moment. Name, date of birth, address, ethnicity, religion, first spoken language and school are essential pieces of information, as are the details of the child's carer.

Establishing who has parental responsibility is vital. Not only can this raise issues regarding private fostering arrangements, but it also has legal implications for consent to medical interventions. Since The Children Act of 1989 parents not only have parental rights but also responsibilities both for and to their children.

Parental responsibility is automatic for the child's birth mother and for the biological father if married to the mother. However, for unmarried fathers parental responsibility is not automatic. It can be granted to the father by the mother or acquired through the court. Parental responsibility can also be shared via the court process by others, for example other members of a family, or indeed by the Local Authority. Parental responsibility is a complicated but necessary piece of information that should be recorded and regarded as of great importance.

The names and contact numbers of other professionals working with the family ought to be clearly identifiable in the child's record. Details of health visitors, social workers or therapists are all vital pieces of information.

A position paper from the Royal College of General Practitioners *The Role of Primary Care in the Protection of Children from Abuse and Neglect* outlines the common indicators pertaining to child abuse that may present in primary health-care.[7] These are grouped under four general headings:

- physical abuse
- emotional abuse
- neglect
- sexual abuse.

Practice nurses need to familiarize themselves with the indicators for each of these four areas as they are just as likely to spot such conditions in their clinical situations as their GP colleagues.

In addition to skilled observation, nurses need to be able to take systematic histories (Box 33.1). A series of questions needs to be asked, and the answers should not only be from the parent but from the child as well, if appropriate. Fraser competency should be taken into account for older children, but be careful that child-protection matters are not masked by applying the Fraser competency rule.[8] Where English is not the first language, consider engaging an interpreter.

Developing practice tools that make gathering patient details and systematic questioning a matter of routine enquiry will help to boost the practice nurse's confidence in taking effective and accurate histories.

SEEKING ADVICE

When PCTs replaced the old health authorities, a letter was sent from the DoH placing the

---

BOX 33.1   Systematic questioning

Ask the patient/parent:

- WHAT is the injury/condition?
- HOW did it happen?
- WHEN did it happen?
- WHERE did it happen?
- WHO was with the child when it happened?
- Do they have parental responsibility?
- WHO brought the child to the surgery?
- Do they have parental responsibility?

Ask yourself:

- Is the explanation consistent with the injury?
- Has there been a delay in reporting?
- Does the explanation change between tellings?
- Is this injury/condition acceptable and reasonable?
- Should I seek advice?

---

responsibility for child-protection practice squarely at the feet of the new organizations. The letter instructed the new Chief Executives of the PCTs to employ child-protection professionals to take the child-protection agenda forward.

Designated nurses and 'named nurses' should be available to offer specialist advice, support and training to practice nurses working with children and families. However, the Royal College of Nursing reports that provision in the UK is patchy, and in reality recruitment of child-protection professionals is problematic.

Sadly, the structures in place may not afford expert child-protection advice and support 24 hours per day 7 days per week. Out-of-hours advice may still need to be sought from Social Services Emergency Duty Teams. Although this advice may not come from a health perspective, it is safer than not seeking advice at all.

In general, the designated nurse role is concerned with the strategic overview and coordination of child-protection practice throughout a geographical or PCT area. Named nurses for child protection are more concerned in the day-to-day

management of casework and practitioner supervision, and are more likely to give practice-based advice.

Practice nurses must find out the support networks and structures for child-protection practice in their PCT area and they should also familiarize themselves with the local Area Child Protection Committee multi-agency procedures and any local child-protection protocols designed for primary healthcare practitioners.

Most areas provide training, either single- or multi-agency, to enable practitioners to practise safely. Child-protection training should be part of every practice nurse's personal development plan.

CONCLUSION

Practice nurses are key practitioners in identifying and referring children in need of support or protection. In order to do this they need to understand the modern child-protection practice drivers and be prepared to take responsibility in this area of work. Support from designated and named nurses for child protection is available in PCTs, and practice nurses should ensure they

---

ESSENTIAL SKILLS

- Find out who your child-protection designated and named nurses are and where they are located
- Include child-protection training in your personal development plan and find out what courses are available
- Locate your child-protection procedures and protocols
- Use routine systematic questioning and recording techniques
- Trust your observations and intuition and always act in the best interest of the child. Ask if you are unsure, challenge if you disagree

know who their child-protection advisers are and how to contact them.

Child protection requires a level of confidence brought about by reflective practice and training, access to advice and the provision of sound practice protocols. If these do not exist then the practice nurse should be able to challenge their senior management structure to bring about change and push child protection higher up the priority list.

Child-protection performance management and competencies will be introduced over the next few years, particularly for primary healthcare professionals. While waiting for these developments to become mainstream we, as primary healthcare practitioners and registered nurses, should strive to ensure that we are never implicated in the mess of poor practice that contributed to the unnecessary death of Victoria Climbié.

REFERENCES

1. Lord Laming (Chairman). The Victoria Climbié Inquiry. London: HMSO, 2003.
2. DFES. Every child matters. Available at: http://www.dfes.gov.uk
3. Department of Health, Department for Education and Employment and Home Office. Working Together to Safeguard Children. London: HMSO, 1999. Available at: http://www.dh.gov.uk
4. Department of Health, Department for Education and Skills, Home Office. What to Do if You're Worried a Child is Being Abused. London: DoH Publications, 2003. Available at: http://www.dh.gov.uk
5. Royal College of Nursing. Child protection: Every Nurses' Responsibility Guidance for Nursing Staff. London: Royal College of Nursing, 2002.
6. Department of Health. The Framework for the Assessment of Children in Need and Their Families. London: DoH, 2002. Available at: http://www.dh.gov.uk
7. Carter YH, Bannon MJ. The Role of Primary Care in the Protection o f Children from Abuse and Neglect. A Position Paper for the Royal College of General Practitioners with Endorsement from the Royal College of Paediatrics and Child Health, the National Society for the Prevention of Cruelty to Children, the British Association of Medical Managers and the NHS Confederation. London: RCGP, 2002. Available at: http://www.rcgp.org.uk
8. Fraser Guidelines. Gillick v West Norfolk and Wisbeach Area Health Authority (1985) 3 All ER 402 (HL).

Chapter 34

Choosing a practice

Sue Nutbrown

Practice nursing can be the most rewarding nursing discipline in primary care. The role has evolved in response to changing health needs and healthcare delivery. Practice nurses have a role in general practice that is complementary to, but distinct from, the role of health visitors and district nurses.

However, as practice nurses are usually employed by GPs and are not managed in the traditional nursing sense, they are effectively working outside the NHS. This has allowed greater freedom to develop the role, but has also led to huge diversity.

Gaining the skills, knowledge and competence needed for practice nursing is a 'Catch 22' situation. In most areas of the country there are no official pre-registration placements with practice nurses. A nurse has to be in a post already to access any relevant post-registration training.

All general practices are part of a primary care organization (PCO); these are the statutory bodies that replaced health authorities and are responsible for delivering healthcare to their local population. In England these are known as primary care trusts (PCTs).

BOARDS AND COMMITTEES

Each PCT has a board responsible to the Strategic Health Authority and ultimately the Secretary of State for the overall performance of the trust. The

PCT Board typically has 11 members: a chairperson, the chief executive and finance director of the PCT, five lay members and three of the professional members of the Professional Executive Committee (PEC).

Much of the day-to-day decision-making and strategic development rests with the PEC. Committee members should be mainly healthcare professionals (up to ten clinicians), with significant representation from general practice. This should be balanced with nurses and other community professionals, public health experts and social services.

GMS OR PMS?

There are two types of general practice: those financed as General Medical Service (GMS) and those financed as Personal Medical Service (PMS). PMS practices have a locally negotiated contract which does not have to be held by a GP. GMS practices have a nationally negotiated contract with the Secretary of State. The new GMS contract means that there is less difference between PMS and GMS, and it opens up new challenges and opportunities for practice nurses.

FINDING THE RIGHT PRACTICE

Every general practice is different. It could be a single-handed or group practice, with or without a branch surgery and perhaps with a dispensing service. Practices also vary by location and patient population, for example a rural or urban area, with an ageing or an ethnically diverse population.

If you are considering a job as a practice nurse you should do some research, visit some practices, talk to the staff, find out about the ethos of the practice, discover how many nurses are employed, how long they have been there and whether or not they would allow you to observe them.

You should find out which consulting room you will be expected to use. Check that it has a couch with screens, a good light, a hand-washing basin and a desk with a networked computer. Also find out if there is a 'panic button' and whether patients can access the room easily.

At interview it is important to find out about any proposed induction programme and any regular meetings held at the practice, and to establish the lines of communication with the district nurses and health visitor.

EMPLOYMENT AND LEGAL ISSUES

The contract of employment starts as soon as you begin work. By law an employee must receive a written statement of the main terms of employment and an indication of disciplinary and grievance procedures within 2 months of starting work.[1] Some of the most important elements in the contract are:

- pay scales, increments, annual reviews and adjustments in line with NHS increases
- study leave entitlement
- sick leave/pay and carer's leave.

All practice nurses should have a job description, which provides the basis for negotiation on pay scales. The RCN document *Guidance on Employing Nurses in General Practice* contains specimen contracts and model disciplinary and grievance procedures.[1] See Box 34.1 for the important aspects that should be covered by a job description. The employer must check the nurse's registration with the Nursing and Midwifery Council (NMC).

INSURANCE

All practice nurses must have their own indemnity insurance. Practices often have a form of group insurance that claims to cover all

---

BOX 34.1   Points to be covered by a job description

- Title of post
- Relationships – who is the post holder accountable to?
- Minimum qualifications required
- Job purpose
- Key areas of responsibility
- Education, training and development opportunities, and responsibilities
- Professional responsibilities
- Date of issue and review date

---

clinicians, but you are advised to check the 'small print' in these policies to ensure that you are fully covered for all the duties you undertake. Some companies insist on extra premiums for nurses who take on extended or expanded roles. Although employers are vicariously liable for the actions and omissions of their employees, registered nurses are 'personally accountable for their practice ... regardless of advice or directions from another professional'.[2]

Patient records

Good record keeping is vital in general practice. Medical records should be shared with all clinicians, whether these are hand written 'Lloyd George' notes or computerized clinical records. If the practice uses a computerized clinical system for all consultations the new practice nurse must attend training sessions before seeing patients.

PROFESSIONAL AND CLINICAL RESPONSIBILITIES

To practise competently, you must possess the knowledge, skills and abilities required for lawful, safe and effective practice without direct supervision. You must acknowledge the limits of your professional competence and only undertake practice and accept responsibilities for those activities in which you are competent.[2]

Most new practice nurses are aware of the limitations of their knowledge and experience but can be put in difficult situations where they are expected to carry out a procedure they are not trained to do. Unfortunately many GPs do not understand that a number of the procedures carried out by nurses every day in general practice are not part of the pre-registration curriculum and need to be acquired after qualifying. A comprehensive training needs analysis must be undertaken when employment commences, and both the employer and the nurse must agree the scope of practice to be undertaken, the training required and how this will be carried out.

Many procedures may not need a formal training course, but the management of some chronic diseases, such as diabetes, asthma and coronary heart disease (CHD), does require specific knowledge and competence.

Clinical protocols are valuable tools that define the areas of responsibility within the practice team (Box 34.2). They enable nurses to develop their skills within an agreed framework and should

---

BOX 34.2   Suggested areas to be covered in a clinical protocol

- Aims and objectives
- Staff requirements
- Patients eligible to attend
- Timings
- Type of assessment/consultation
- Referral system
- Follow-up review
- Documentation
- Evaluation/audit
- Date of protocol review/update

Source: MDU. Protocols and the practice nurse. J Med Def Union 1998; 14: 21.

allow for clinical judgement. Protocols should be written and agreed by all team members.

CONTINUING PROFESSIONAL DEVELOPMENT

All nurses are required to comply with two PREP (post-registration education and practice) standards:

- The PREP (practice) standard – you must have worked in some capacity by virtue of your nursing, midwifery or health visiting qualification during the previous 5 years for a minimum of 100 days (750 hours).
- The PREP (CPD) standard – you must undertake at least 5 days or 35 hours of learning activity relevant to your work during the 3 years prior to your renewal of registration, you must maintain a personal professional profile of your learning activity and comply with any request from the NMC to audit how you have met these requirements.

A Personal Development Plan (PDP) helps with identifying the learning activities needed to comply with the PREP CPD standard. It can be used as the basis of discussions in annual reviews/appraisal.

New practice nurses should agree to a review 3 months after starting in the role and to an annual appraisal/review. These are times when skills gaps are identified, learning objectives are set and a learning programme agreed. It should also be noted that the practice team may require the nurse to learn new skills in order to develop services.

Ideally new practice nurses should have a period of preceptorship with an experienced nurse. Many PCTs have employed professional development nurses who may be able to arrange this. Following on from this all practice nurses should be involved in clinical supervision. This is defined as: 'a formal process of professional support and learning which enables individual practitioners to develop knowledge and compe-

tence, assume responsibility for their own practice and enhance consumer protection and safety of care'.[3]

Clinical supervision enables nurses to discuss their work regularly with another experienced health professional. It involves reflecting on practice in order to learn from experience and improve competence. It is recommended that a minimum of 1 hour a month is allocated for supervision.

CLINICAL GOVERNANCE

Clinical governance is defined as:

> *A framework through which NHS organisations are accountable for continuously improving the quality of their services and safeguarding high standards of care by creating an environment in which excellence in clinical care will flourish.*[4]

Most practice nurses are the lead in their practice for infection control and many have health and safety remits (risk management). All PCTs should have a process in place for dealing with any concerns you may have about colleagues (e.g. managing poor performance).

Clinical governance is about every member of staff recognizing his or her role in the whole team's provision of high-quality care.

CONCLUSION

Primary care is changing to deliver the NHS Plan. There are many challenges and opportunities for practice nurses. As those more experienced take on new roles and responsibilities, new practice nurses must be encouraged to enter the profession.

The new GMS contract promotes skill mix and will encourage the development of career frameworks for practice nurses. However this requires training programmes, development opportunities and support networks.

REFERENCES

1. RCN. Guidance on Employing Nurses in General Practice. London: RCN, 2000.
2. NMC. Code of Professional Conduct. London: NMC, 2002.
3. NHSE. A Vision for the Future – The Nursing, Midwifery and Health Visiting Contribution to Health and Healthcare. London: DoH, 1993.
4. Department of Health. A First Class Service. Health Service Circular 1998/113. London: DoH, 1998.

FURTHER READING

Tettersall M, Sawyer J, Salisbury C. Handbook of Practice Nursing. Edinburgh: Churchill Livingston, 1997.

Macdougald N, King P, Jones A, Eveleigh M. A Toolkit for Practice Nurses. Chichester: Aeneas Press, 2001.

RCN. Good Practice in Infection Control. London: RCN, 2001.

ICNA. Infection Control Guidance for General Practice. Available from: Fitwise, Tel. 01506 811077.

Roland MD, Baker R. Handbook: Clinical Governance a Practical Guide for Primary Care Teams. Manchester: University of Manchester, 1999. Available at: http://www.npcrdc.man.ac.uk

Rughani A. The GP's Guide to Personal Development Plans. Oxford: Radcliffe Medical Press, 2000.

Chapter 35

General practice: the NHS – the practice nurse

Simon Ebbett

Traditionally, general practice has held two key roles in the NHS, that of the health service's gatekeeper and that of the patient's advocate. It also increasingly has a public health role.

General practice is a blizzard of bewildering acronyms. The important ones are listed and defined in Box 35.1.

GATEKEEPER TO THE NHS

The gatekeeper role is sorting the wheat from the chaff, or deciding whom to refer for tests or to hospital/specialist care, whom to manage within primary care and whom to tell to go home and let the illness sort itself out. The key to this is recognizing clinical alarm bells when they go off, which some GPs say is the art of the job. As a result, GPs often talk about risk: the decision about whether to play a waiting game and see if a patient's condition resolves itself, or to make a referral which could turn out to waste everybody's time and money and unnecessarily worry the patient.

While the gatekeeper role is, in theory, based on clinical factors, the GP also partly performs a cost-control task. By controlling access to diagnostic services and secondary and tertiary care, the practice cuts unnecessary NHS spending and prevents waiting lists and times blowing out.

Hence the never-ending spats between hospitals, GPs and trusts over referring behaviour: consultants say GPs make their lives hell with constant pointless referrals, GPs say the hospitals never appreciate what practices protect them from.

The advent of community matrons could change this as, under current plans, GPs will no longer exclusively be the gatekeepers. Community matrons are to get powers to order diagnostic investigations and refer. As yet, it is unclear how much GP input there will be to such decisions. The community matron plan illustrates the Government's growing focus on public health, and most of the work involved, such as screening and checks, is pushed onto practices and subsequently nurses.

PATIENTS' ADVOCATE

The practice is also the patient's advocate. It is the central hub and starting point of a patient's dealings with the NHS, save for a trip to A&E or a GUM clinic. The practice builds often life-long relationships with patients, compared with hospital staff, who meet a patient perhaps only once or twice.

BOX 35.1   The important acronyms used in general practice

- **GMS** General medical services – refers to the contract that most practices work under, otherwise known as nGMS or GMS2, as it is the second version of this contract

- **PMS** Personal medical services – an alternative contract, which about 40% of GPs work under

- **PCO** Primary care organization – body that carries out NHS management at the local level and has all the money. In England they are called primary care trusts (PCTs), in Scotland and Northern Ireland they are health boards, and in Wales they are local health boards (LHBs)

- **PEC** Professional Executive Committee – committee on an English PCT that represents doctors, nurses and other professionals and which advises the trust

- **SHA** Strategic Health Authority – the next level up from a PCO in NHS management and the body that controls PCOs and secondary care trusts in a region (sometimes written as StHA)

- **DH** or **DoH** Department of Health – each of the four nations of the UK has its own department, and in Northern Ireland its title is Department of Health, Social Services and Public Safety (DHSSPS)

- **BMA** British Medical Association – the trade union for doctors. GPs are represented nationally by its General Practitioners Committee (GPC) and locally by Local Medical Committees (LMCs)

- **GMC** General Medical Council – the body that holds the medical register and regulates doctors. It can strike off doctors. The GMC also produces guidance to doctors on the standards, behaviours and actions expected of them

- **RCGP** Royal College of General Practitioners – sets GPs' education criteria and standards for clinical practice

- **NPSA** National Patient Safety Agency – body to which doctors and nurses can anonymously report adverse incidents. The information is used to spot trends and share data rather than discipline practitioners

- **NCAA** National Clinical Assessment Authority – body to which doctors and nurses can whistle-blow about a colleague. It can investigate doctors

The practice will often act on behalf of the patient, pushing for them to get onto a waiting list, explaining the results and implications of tests and treatments, managing chronic conditions and repeat prescriptions, and dealing with the patient as a rounded person and not just as a clinical condition or a slot on an operating schedule.

This relationship is considered to be one of the most rewarding aspects of primary care. But it also causes conflicts, when the practice has to challenge or deny a patient while at the same time trying not to harm the overall relationship. A classic example is the act of writing a sick note to explain work absence, a role practices do not want and a source of endless run-ins between doctors, patients and employers.

Allied to this advocate role is the concept of 'continuity of care', or the practice knowing the patient and their history, and making decisions based not just on clinical factors but also on their knowledge of that individual. Many consider this to be in jeopardy because of the increasing fragmentation of primary care.

The practice also holds patients' medical records, and GPs take the duty of guarding patients' confidentiality very seriously. They see the NHS's current £6.2 billion IT overhaul as a massive threat to this, as it will put records on a central database and open access to other doctors, nurses and health professionals.

General practice has a third, unofficial role within the NHS – that of the health service's dump. The result of most policy initiatives or lobby group demands, regardless of the subject at hand, is some new task assigned to general practice. There will also almost inevitably be a suggestion that GPs get more training in whatever particular clinical area is being addressed, which has most doctors hitting the roof.

General practice also cops the fallout of the health scares that dominate the press each week. When a big news story breaks about a drug or condition, practices expect a wave of anxious patients demanding information and reassurance. Typically, primary care will have had little warning or guidance, and so will resort to trying to find a copy of that day's newspaper to find out what the patients are talking about. Your first port of call should be the *Daily Mail*, which revels in medical horror stories.

CONTRACTUAL RELATIONSHIP WITH THE NHS

Traditionally, a general practice has been a small business, run by self-employed doctors who contract their services to the NHS. The GPs run the practice as partners, with ultimate responsibility for management, financial and clinical/medico-legal matters. They take shares of the practice's profits. A very small number of practices have made nurses, pharmacists and practice managers partners.

The 'independent contractor' status is a source of pride to GPs. While it gives them a great deal of freedom in running their practices as they want, its big benefit has been having the independence to challenge health bosses in a way that being employed by the NHS would not allow. It also has tax advantages. This is arguably a slightly false construct, given that the NHS is a monopoly and practices are heavily subsidized for costs such as staff and premises.

For a practice nurse, it means that, instead of being an NHS employee, you are usually an employee of the practice. Unlike in hospital, where the doctor is a colleague who leads the clinical team but has little other authority, the GP is the practice nurse's boss.

This puts practice nurses outside of the NHS pay scales and employment terms and conditions, but in reality most GPs take their lead from the NHS, and practices are encouraged to adhere to Agenda for Change (AfC). Some do not but, as business people, most GPs realize that if they do not match AfC, they simply will not get the staff.

At a local level, NHS management takes the form of the primary care organization (PCO). In England, they are primary care trusts (PCTs), in Scotland and Northern Ireland they are health boards, and in Wales they are local health boards (LHBs).

The PCO covers a geographical area and holds all the money. All the practices in the area contract their services to the PCO, which also commissions other community-based care and some hospital care, and sets many of the local spending priorities and clinical guidelines.

In recent years, an increasing number of nurses has been employed by the PCO, which then places them in practices. A PCO-employed nurse comes under AfC.

English PCTs are run by boards, with input from a professional executive committee (PEC) – a group of local doctors, nurses and other health professionals that advises the trust and makes some policy decisions. The PEC chairman will usually be a GP.

The extent to which the PEC has any true authority varies from trust to trust. Similarly, the relationships between practices and their PCOs range from harmonious and efficient joint working to mutual distrust and constant conflict.

The trust's financial position and competence can have a direct effect on the quality and range of services available locally. If a PCO is debt-ridden, practices will get few chances to innovate or provide particular services, and the organization will put pressure on cutting costs in such areas as prescribing.

THE MEDICO-LEGAL REALM

Generally speaking, there are two areas in which practice nurses can get into medico-legal difficulty: a failure to meet the terms of their own or their practice's contract, and negligence.

In the first case, the nurse will undergo a disciplinary process. This will be within the practice if the practice employs the nurse, or through the PCO if that is the employer. In negligence cases, the liability of the nurse and the GP(s) involved depends on the case. Where the practice has provided nurses with clear and

appropriate protocols and the nurse fails to follow them, or the nurse makes a mistake which any similarly qualified and experienced nurse should not be expected to make, then the nurse will probably be solely liable.

If a GP has delegated a task to a nurse but has not taken reasonable steps to ensure that the nurse is competent, or to ensure that he or she has appropriate resources (e.g. time, training, assistance, protocols), the liability may be shared. It is worth remembering that, regardless of anyone else's liability, nurses must observe the limits of their own competence. To clarify any areas of misunderstanding, only the nurse will be answerable in any Nursing and Midwifery Council (NMC) proceedings.

Complaints against a practice go through a number of possible procedures. A patient can complain directly to the practice or to the PCO. The trust will aim to resolve the complaint at that level but, if it cannot, then it must set up an independent review panel to investigate and rule on the matter. If the panel feels the subject is too serious, or has been unable to resolve it, then it will refer the nurse involved to the NMC, or the doctor to the General Medical Council (GMC). The GMC is the doctor equivalent of the NMC, and has the power to strike a doctor off the medical register.

Patients can also refer a complaint to the Health Service Ombudsman, if they are unsatisfied with the outcome of local procedures. If the Ombudsman decides to investigate the complaint further, he or she can order action to be taken, and general reports of these investigations are published.

Adverse incident reporting and whistle-blowing are increasingly encouraged in general practice. The National Patient Safety Agency (NPSA) handles adverse incident reporting, and does so on a strictly anonymous basis. Its aim is to identify trends, correct system weaknesses and educate practitioners to prevent future incidents.

The National Clinical Assessment Authority (NCAA) handles whistle-blowing about a specific practitioner, but encourages alerts to be made to the PCO first. Many moves have been made in recent years to ensure the NHS protects whistle-blowers.

The medico-legal side of general practice is about to undergo massive change. This is a result of the actions of mass murderer Harold Shipman and, to a much lesser extent, former Kent GP Clifford Ayling, who sexually assaulted many patients over a 20-year period. The Shipman Inquiry has recommended widespread changes and the Government is currently reviewing the GMC's role, which could possibly close the body.

As a result of the Ayling case, practice nurses may have to act as chaperones for GPs in any intimate examination, although a decision has not yet been made on this.

MEDICO-POLITICAL BODIES

Doctors are represented by the British Medical Association (BMA), the profession's trade union. Within the BMA, general practice matters are handled by the General Practitioners Committee (GPC). The GPC represents the profession in negotiations with the Government and makes public statements.

At a local level, Local Medical Committees (LMCs) effectively act as branch offices of the GPC, representing GPs in negotiations and disputes with PCOs or other local bodies. They also provide guidance and political representation at that level. LMCs are made up of GPs, with some administration support, with the LMC chairman and the secretary performing the most public roles. A practice which has a GP in one of these roles receives a lot of press calls.

General GP attitudes towards the BMA and its subsidiaries vary from vague apathy to outright hostility. A vocal minority of doctors believe the association is too soft and too cosy with the Government and has sold the profession out, while many others do not pay that much attention to medico-politics and keep paying BMA membership fees simply to get the *British Medical Journal* for free.

Chapter 36

The type of contract your practice has with the NHS will affect your role

Simon Ebbett

CHAPTER CONTENTS

In many ways, general practice is all about contracts. The type of contract a practice has with the NHS often affects how the GPs work and can explain why a question about PMS is probably not a comment about your mood! This chapter explains these contracts and looks at what the future may hold.

CONTRACTS

Until 1998, practices had little choice about the type of contract they could sign with the NHS. It was the old general medical services (GMS) deal, otherwise known as the Red Book. This deal was effectively imposed on general practice in 1990 and was roundly despised.

Under this old GMS contract, practices were paid both according to the number of patients on their lists, and through a bewildering and bureaucratic system of item-of-service payments, together with clinical targets and incentives. As the contract contained no effective mechanism for controlling a practice's workload, it was referred to as the John Wayne contract, as in: 'A GP's gotta do what a GP's gotta do'. It is still blamed in large part for the recruitment crisis that hit general practice in the 1990s.

In April 2004, a new GMS contract came into effect. This will be outlined below, but in short its aims were to cut bureaucracy, control workload and reward quality care.

Personal medical services

In 1998, before the new GMS contract was negotiated, the Government approved an alternative arrangement to the Red Book called personal medical services (PMS), and the first wave of PMS pilots started in 1999. Under this PMS contract practices work out the services they want to provide and the staff and other costs they need to meet, and agree a contract negotiated between themselves and the primary care organization (PCO). The latter then makes a single monthly payment. The aim of PMS was to encourage innovation, and allow practices to prioritize and design care based on local needs, and to offer an alternative to the Red Book's bureaucracy. It also allowed GPs and nurses to set up specialized services, for example practices that solely treat the homeless, drug addicts and/or asylum seekers and refugees. PMS also allowed for the contractor to be someone other than a GP, and there are a few nurse-led practices. The Government also introduced PMS Plus, which gives extra money for practices wanting to expand their staff or premises.

The first practices to go to PMS did so in its spirit of innovation, but GPs have increasingly turned to PMS solely to get more money and/or escape the bureaucracy of the old GMS. By April 2004, 40% of English practices were on PMS contracts. The Government has never allowed GPs' national representatives to negotiate on behalf of PMS doctors, saying such contracts are between the practice and the PCO, which has led to fears about the erosion of GPs' collective bargaining power at a national level.

Increasingly, many GPs are taking jobs as salaried doctors, i.e. employees of either the practice or the PCO. The attraction of this, particularly for young GPs, is the lack of responsibility for the practice's financial and management aspects, allowing them to focus on clinical matters and leave work at work at the end of the day. It also means they do not have to buy into the practice, saving them the burden of a second mortgage or hefty loan early in their careers. Many young GPs also spend time as locums before settling down, while others work under the NHS' flexible careers scheme, which allows them to work fewer hours or return from an extended absence.

The introduction of the new GMS contract (see below) brought with it other contractual options. The first of these is PCT medical services (PCTMS) which is a PCT-owned and managed health centre. Another is alternative provider medical services (APMS), where the PCO contracts someone other than a GMS or PMS GP practice to provide particular services. Typically, the provider will be a private company specializing in an area of care or possibly a pharmacy. This has opened general practice to competition and created a market for PCOs. It is still early days for both PCTMS and APMS, and a clear picture of their impact has yet to emerge.

THE NEW GMS CONTRACT

The new GMS contract brought in some of the biggest changes to primary care since the NHS was created in 1948 and has affected all practices regardless of their contractual status.

As outlined above, GPs hated the old GMS contract. In 2001 they voted to enter negotiations for a new GMS deal, which came into effect in April 2004. Despite voting overwhelmingly to accept the new contract, GPs have done little but complain about it ever since. While the old contract was called the Red Book, the new deal is mostly referred to as nGMS or GMS2.

The contract's structure is aimed at defining and controlling workload. It is separated into two areas: core services and enhanced services.

Core services

By default, practices must provide core services. These are split into essential services, which is basically treating the newly ill and terminally ill, and additional services, which are cervical cytology and child health, immunizations, and managing chronic conditions. Practices can opt out of additional services if they can prove they do not have the staff or partners to do the work, but must go through a lengthy process to do so and lose a lot of money. For providing these services, the practice receives a monthly lump sum payment that is based on factors such as their list size, the age of their patients, and the nature of the area (i.e. how poor it is or how rural). This was designed to remove the bureaucracy and multiple funding streams of the Red Book.

Enhanced services

Enhanced services are those that the practice does not provide by default and can choose whether to do so or not. These range from influenza immunization, to specialized alcohol and drug addiction treatment, to minor surgery and minor injury care. The aim of this was to allow practices to either cut their workload or to ensure they were paid for work they had previously been doing for free. The contract places the burden on the PCO to ensure services are available in its area, rather than on individual practices to provide them. Enhanced services enable a GP or a nurse to exercise a particular clinical interest they may have and to bring additional money into the practice.

To do enhanced services work the practice must tender to the PCO for the particular contract. Practices are increasingly competing against others, such as pharmacists and private providers, for the work. PMS practices are also allowed to compete for enhanced services work.

Possibly the biggest change the contract has made to doctors' lives is to remove their 24-hour responsibility for their patients. From January 2005 they could opt out of providing out-of-hours cover and hand that responsibility to the PCO.

Quality and outcomes framework

One key aim of the contract was to reward practices for providing quality care. With this in mind, the contract contains a quality and outcomes framework (QOF), which has a number of targets, both clinical and organizational. Practices earn varying numbers of points for each target they achieve, which translates into money on top of their monthly lump sum.

The QOF is the area of the contract that most affects practice nurses, as they do much of the work involved, such as blood pressure measurements. It is also where a well-organized and efficient practice can make money.

Controversies

There are still a number of controversies around the GMS contract. Many GPs are unhappy with the formula used to calculate the monthly payments, saying it sells short inner-city practices and those working with student populations. The out-of-hours handover has created problems in some areas.

Many GPs also dislike the QOF, saying it has turned them from clinicians into data collectors who tick boxes. The evidence base for some QOF targets has also shifted, and a review has started that will change some targets in 2006. PCTs have also been accused of failing to spend enough money on enhanced services, meaning practices have either had to provide services for free or have been unable to apply for well-paying contracts.

Possibly the biggest controversy has been over the contract's promised function of cutting and defining practices' workloads. In many areas, practices and PCOs have been unable to agree what their core services are. For some, this has led to practices turning away patients wanting treatment such as suture removal or wound dressings, while others have done the work unpaid. GP leaders have failed to help as they refused the profession's request to produce a definitive list of the care they must provide.

THE FUTURE

In addition to standing in the shadow of Harold Shipman (Box 36.1), general practice is undergoing some of the biggest changes it has ever faced. The workforce is undergoing a complete facelift, with the stereotype of the white, middle-aged male family doctor quickly becoming out of date.

The workforce, particularly at the younger end, is increasingly female and ethnically diverse. It also comes from a generation that wants more out of life than 12 hours a day at the surgery followed by a night on-call. Many female doctors prefer to take half- or part-time posts or work flexibly while raising a family. This is one factor in general practice's workforce crisis. The current

---

BOX 36.1   The shadow of Shipman

Harold Frederick Shipman, a GP at Market Street in Hyde, was convicted at Preston Crown Court on 31 January 2000 of 15 murders and of one count of forging a will. He was sentenced to life imprisonment and has since committed suicide in custody.

It is difficult to overestimate the impact Harold Shipman has had on general practice. Two separate inquiries have found that he killed at least 215 people, and possibly 250, with injected diamorphine. Invariably his victims were elderly women who were found dead shortly after a home visit from Shipman.

The impact of this case was felt first in the area of medical regulation. Following Shipman's conviction, the then Health Secretary Alan Milburn came close to scrapping the General Medical Council, saying the practice of doctors regulating themselves had failed to protect patients from a serial killer.

In the years since Shipman's conviction, the GMC and other professional bodies have worked on reforms, but rarely without controversy. Many doctors and members of the public now have little faith in the GMC. Following a report from the Shipman Inquiry in December 2004, which heavily criticized the GMC and its plans for reform, the Government is now reviewing medical regulation, including the role of the Council. This has been the biggest reform of medical regulation in 150 years.

Britain has also seen both an increase in medical scandals and an increasing willingness by the media and the public to assume the worst.

In the months immediately after Shipman's conviction, two GPs were arrested on suspicion of murder following patient deaths. Both were later released without charges, but not before appearing on front pages under somewhat hysterical headlines. The eagerness of police and health bosses to charge in 'to catch another Shipman', before establishing the facts, worried the profession. These were the first of several high-profile scandals in recent years as, in the eyes of the media, doctors shifted from being a pillar of the community to a legitimate target.

The profession's image with the general public has also changed for the worse. Doctors still rate highly in public opinion polls, but that trust and confidence is not as solid as it was, and patients are quicker to question and doubt their GP.

That is perhaps Shipman's biggest legacy. In betraying his own patients' trust, he made the public question their faith in doctors. He proved to them that the unthinkable – a doctor murdering patients – could actually happen.

thinking is that it takes two new GPs to replace each retiring GP.

More and more GPs are taking salaried posts, meaning that future practices will increasingly be PCO-owned and managed, making practice nurses employees of the NHS rather than of independent small businesses.

The nature of general practice and its role in the NHS is also changing. Much more care is being delegated out of hospitals and into the community, largely to improve access for patients. The new GMS contract, when it works as it is supposed to, opens up the opportunity for practices to diversify their work and provide specialized care.

A word becoming increasingly common in general practice is 'gypsies', which has nothing to do with people of Romany extraction and everything to do with GPs with special interests, or GPwSIs.

Allied to this are the growing opportunities for nurses to take on nurse practitioner roles, have prescribing powers, run specialized clinics and become community matrons managing chronic diseases.

By opening the door to private and alternative providers and by creating roles such as community matrons, the Government is also changing the essence of a general practice.

The increasing fragmentation of primary care means the days of the practice being the first port of call and hub of the patient's dealings with the NHS are ending. The practice may no longer be the gatekeeper or the advocate, but just one of the destinations on the journey. Many GPs are worried this means an end to continuity of care and the days of being the patient's own doctor; others says these concepts have never truly mattered anyway.

Index